The Four Paths To

Ultimate Wellness

Revised

Renée Alleyne, Ph.D.

(formerly Renée Parks, Ph.D.)

ISBN-13: 978-1467925259
ISBN-10: 146792525X

Cover Photography: Tarik Jones
Cover Design: Raslikestodraw
Author Photo: Tarik Jones

Reflections on *The Four Paths To Ultimate Wellness*:

The Four Paths To Ultimate Wellness is a sensitive self-reflection of a personal spiritual journey. Renée reveals her own spiritual struggle and growth in such a way that the reader can find comfort, direction, and hope. This is a practical, easy-to-read guide for all of us, young and old, who are seeking to balance mind, body, soul and space.

> Donna Shannon, Ph.D., Pastoral Counselor

The Four Paths To Ultimate Wellness offers us a fresh set of eyes on the age-old question "How do I heal myself?" Renée's firsthand accounts of her own journey in life connects well with the reader, and gives strength in knowing we can all work toward healing ourselves. The suggestions on how to work through the daily challenge of balancing our lives are practical and can be easily applied to busy lifestyles. This book is a must-read for anyone interested in improving their own life and health, and the lives of each one we touch. We are all in this together.

> Bill Pedro, friend in Feng Shui

The Four Paths To Ultimate Wellness sets the tone for healing. The reading paves the way and opens the mind for our life's journey. An amazing work!

> Paulette Williams, Greenbaum Cancer Center

This book is dedicated to my mother, C. Anita Bowen, for it is through her struggle that I found my strength.

Table of Contents

Introduction

The doctor of the future will give no medicine but will interest his patients in the care of the human frame, in diet, and in the cause and prevention of disease.
~Thomas Edison

The United States is the only wealthy, industrialized nation that does not have a universal healthcare system. In 2006, approximately 47 million Americans were without health insurance. Per the National Center for Health Statistics, the United States spends twice as much on healthcare per capita than any other country. From 2000–2006, healthcare premiums accelerated 87%, which may explain why half of bankruptcy filings are the result of medical expenses.

Seventy-five percent of all healthcare dollars are spent on chronic illnesses, including diabetes, obesity, hypertension, lung disease and cancer. Despite the vast number of resources spent on healthcare within the last 30 years, new cases of breast cancer, depression and other chronic illness have been on the rise. The unprecedented acceleration of these conditions has fueled a growing interest in holistic medicine, where one not only treats the symptoms of illness, but considers the patient's lifestyle and emotional well-being.

We are coming to understand that wellness is not just about the body or life circumstances; it is about the consciousness of wholeness in which we live our daily lives. Hospitals, medical professionals, and pharmaceutical companies alike are becoming more open to alternative means that complement traditional healing methods.

I was asked to speak about a holistic approach to wellness at a University of Maryland Medical System, Greenbaum Cancer Center, Center for Image Renewal Breast Cancer Awareness event. I thought long and hard about whether or not I would be the right person for the engagement because I have never had cancer. I felt that a person who had experienced the debilitating disease could better relate to the women. When I began to ponder the idea, the following questions came to me: What could I say to these women? How will I relate to them? What is the life-changing message that I can share to help them transform their lives? What will make them feel better? What will make them feel beautiful?

What ultimately emerged is an incredibly unique holistic approach to wellness coupled with ancient time-tested spiritual wisdom. The book that you are reading flowed on to paper as I wept with compassion for these women. As I wrote, it occurred to me that while most wellness practitioners address the mind, body and soul, a particularly important component was being overlooked. The environment that we live and work in impacts our lives, but it is rarely considered as part of the holistic wellness equation. The space we live in is often the underlying culprit of our ills and the missing link to modern medicine. It also holds the key to the prevention of cancer, heart disease and other chronic diseases.

After writing this book, I was led to create the Wellness Makeover Program, a transformational program for women facing chronic illness, which helps them to explore complementary healing methods to further support their doctor's care. This program teaches how to improve one's well-being and positive self-image by addressing the connection between the mind, body, soul, and spatial surroundings. The positive feedback we received from the participants of the program made it clear to me that this holistic approach to wellness needed to be shared on a global level.

When I speak about a holistic approach to wellness, I am not merely talking about curing symptoms, but rather resolving the root-cause of our ailments. Healing is not a one-size-fits-all undertaking, and we must all decide what works best for us as an individual rather than depend on people, circumstances, or some magical coincidence to save us. Even medicine is rooted in the understanding of how nature works, but some people believe in pharmaceuticals more than our natural healing potential.

Ultimate wellness is a state of consciousness that results in a healthy lifestyle. It starts with a conscious choice to be well and then doing the things that contribute to good health and well-being. This book includes time-tested principles and ancient wisdom that have helped me to feel good and maintain a youthful appearance.

The first section of the book explores potential sources of imbalance and provides ways to improve the way that you feel. The second section provides a few tips and practical solutions that you can easily apply to your life. If you earnestly apply these principles and techniques, you will not only see an extraordinary shift towards optimal health, but you will never look at life in the same way ever again.

PART ONE

The Terrain - Our Spiritual Beliefs

God doesn't ask you to convert yourself. She doesn't ask you to chop off your intellect and believe in faith. She makes a far simpler request. Just stop judging, stop finding fault, stop imposing your expectations, your will, your interruptions, your pictures of reality, and see what happens. ~ Paul Ferrini

I have exhausted countless hours and many sleepless nights in search of the meaning of life and have encountered many spiritual paths. As a young girl, I attended Catholic school but do not have any fond memories to share with you about Catholicism. I vaguely remember a nun here and a priest there, the repeated kneeling and standing during Mass and ironing the pleats in my grade-school uniform.

Fast-forward to my adult life where I experienced many years in various sects of Christianity. I have heard hundreds of sermons and talks and attended countless churches and spiritual centers in search of the perfect place for my spiritual growth. I enjoyed the preachers who had a colorful style and brought life to ancient biblical stories; but if I am honest about it, I cannot say that I wholeheartedly embraced the Christian belief system.

I remember the days when I read the Bible from cover to cover because I wanted to know everything God said. I must admit that much of what was contained within the pages of my leather-bound Bible was rather unsettling.

While there was definitely lots of good life-lesson material, all the killing and hatred among the cast of characters appalled me.

I made attempts at memorizing as much of the scriptures as possible so that I could recite passages and quote where they were in the Bible. This was my idea of being a good Christian. While I earnestly wanted to do right by God, religion was in my head but not in my heart.

I also discovered that many people, including preachers, were quoting scripture that could not be found in the Bible. When I tried to find quotes like: "God looks out for babies and fools," "God works in mysterious ways" and "money is the root of all evil," they were nowhere to be found.

The mixed messages that I received in the traditional church were very confusing and caused me to search even more deeply. The duality of a loving God that gave us free will to do whatever we wanted but could be vengeful enough to kill those who did not meet impossible demands was a hard pill to swallow. It sounded more like a diagnosis for bipolar disorder than the God who made the heavens, the earth and everything in between. If God oversaw everything, how could anything happen that He didn't permit? Things just were not adding up for me.

I also had trouble embracing the idea that the world was going to end, since this story had been told for so many years but had never actually happened. This looming thought was not only contrary to my beliefs; it was depressing and offered me little hope for the future.

I was well versed in all of the spiritual jargon; I could talk the talk but was unable to walk the walk. It was unbelievably hard to be a "good Christian" because it meant that I was not able to associate with anyone who wasn't of the same faith or, as the preacher said, "equally yoked." This eliminated practically everyone in my social circle and workplace. Other religions were considered a "cult" because they chose to call God by a different name. Sex was forbidden before marriage, and so I married simply to avoid feeling the guilt. My world was closing in on me and all the demands that Christianity placed on me were too much for me to handle. No matter what I did to try to appease God as a Christian, I would always be a sinner and never truly worthy of His love.

Despite all the searching that I had done, nothing seemed to heal my wounds and I was hurting inside. In my late 30s, I began my search for answers outside of the church. I absorbed all the spiritual information that I could find like a sponge. A co-worker introduced me to *A Course in Miracles* that was taught by Marianne Williamson. I became a student of the course and listened to countless cassette tapes. One of the most life-changing ideas that I discovered was, "Nothing real can be threatened and nothing unreal exists. Herein lies the peace of God." This helped me to understand that much of what I was unhappy about was what I made up in my mind and was what the course referred to as an illusion.

The Course also helped me to understand how romantic relationships could be destructive, particularly when I reserved my love only for that "special" person. These new concepts were quite challenging to apply consistently but things did seem to start making more sense and I was marginally feeling better about my life.

In my early 40s, I became ill due to serious problems with fibroid tumors lodged in the wall of my womb, and major surgery was necessary. In preparation to convalesce; I went to the library for reading material. One of the books that I found on CD was called *Conversations with God* by Neale Donald Walsh. The idea of having a conversation with God was a little unsettling but the title made me very curious, so I checked the CDs out of the library and tucked them into my overnight bag.

After my surgery, I was scheduled to be in the hospital for several days. As the time went by, I slowly recovered from the deep incision that stretched across my lower abdomen. While lying across the hospital bed, I felt that this was a good time to listen to *Conversations with God*. After a few minutes of listening, it almost felt as if I had died and gone to heaven. I was a little drugged up and remember opening my eyes a few times because I could not remember where I was.

The voice on the CD was so comforting that it seemed as if God himself was speaking directly to me. Prior to hearing the CD, I always saw myself as being outside of God. Hearing the messages that Walsh conveyed in his book changed my whole idea about God. Finally, there was someone who understood how isolated I was feeling! I began to feel more connected and a part of God, and I realized that if I was a part of God, then there was nothing that I needed to do to be accepted by Him. This was a very healing experience that led me in a new and exciting direction on my spiritual journey.

After my experience with *Conversations with God*, I lost interest in traditional Christianity. I stopped going to Sunday services and packed my Bible away. Feeling as if I was in a spiritual limbo, it was a welcome invitation when my sister suggested that I attend a Unity church service with her. She had been attending services there for a while and felt that it might be something that I would also enjoy. The people in the congregation were very friendly and seemed sincere. The smiles, hugs, and laughter that filled the Unity Center were very warm and appealing.

The message was much more palatable and in line with what I knew in my heart to be the truth. I learned that Unity honors all religions and respects everyone's right to choose his or her own spiritual path. I eventually joined that church and was a member there for several years.

While attending Unity, I was still very eager to learn as much as possible about anything that might continue to support me in my spiritual journey. Quite by accident, my boss at the time, thinking that I was a Buddhist, gave me a book on Feng Shui (pronounced *fung schway*). Feng Shui is a philosophy developed thousands of years ago in China that reveals how to balance the energies of any given space to assure good health and good fortune. I became fascinated with the idea that our surrounding space could influence us in these ways. I wasn't 100% sure Feng Shui would work for me but I was open and willing to try something new.

Soon after reading the Feng Shui book, I hired a seasoned Feng Shui practitioner to support me with the renovation I was making to a rental property I owned. Within a very short time of making the suggested adjustments to my space, my rental property went from having no tenants to being fully and prosperously occupied. The concepts that I learned during my consultation were so powerful and undeniably effective that I decided to learn as much as I could about it so that I could teach others about this amazing gift. I completed a Feng Shui apprenticeship program and began performing Feng Shui consultations nationally and teaching classes about this new-found gift. More details about Feng Shui are covered in Part II of this book.

There was an overwhelming response from the Feng Shui class that I taught at the Unity Center and was invited to teach a Feng Shui class for a spiritual center close to my home. I knew that this center taught "Religious Science" and "Science of Mind," but I was unfamiliar with this teaching. To get a better feel for the people that I'd be teaching, I decided to attend a Sunday service. As soon as I set foot in the center, I was warmly welcomed by a greeter who gave me a big childlike smile and a huge hug. I enjoyed the message and felt so welcomed and that I returned to the center and for the next few years I studied Religious Science.

I learned that Religious Science is a philosophy that integrates spiritual truths with science and physics. One of the core beliefs of Religious Science is that we are all one and part of the One Mind. Our intentions and ideas flow through a field of consciousness, which affects and creates the world around us. In other words, "as we think, so we become." The classes that I attended were life-changing and taught me that the secret to living a successful and healthy life is to consciously choose positive and productive thoughts. I soon began to consistently engage in prayer, meditation, affirmations, and the practice of watching my thought patterns. It was not long before I saw dramatic, positive changes in my life. I was generally much happier and was doing a better job of coping with the ups and downs of life.

To better support my friends, family and clients with the principles that changed my life, I decided to pursue a doctoral degree in Holistic Life Coaching with the International Metaphysical Ministry. Their program covered a wide range of mystical topics that were like the teachings of Religious Science. This experience deepened my daily spiritual practices and my connection with a loving God. After many years of searching, the concepts of hell-and-damnation and fire-and-brimstone were replaced with a world I could connect with, full of positive possibilities.

Ernest Holmes, founder of Religious Science, wrote "Healing is not a process but a revelation; for the revealing of the perfect man always heals." My healing revelation was that we are already perfect in the eyes of God and that we need no salvation for His approval. My closed mind and judgment towards people who did not practice my faith blossomed into openness towards all people. I can embrace the idea that there is only one God and that we are all connected, and in so doing, my pain eased, and my soul healed.

We are more alike than we are different. We all breathe the same air and have warm blood running through our veins. We drink the same water and need food for our existence. We all need shelter and clothing for our bodies. Yet, Sunday mornings have been the most segregated hour for centuries. I have learned to respect what a person believes because no one religion has a franchise on God. If there was only one path to God, everyone who practiced that faith would have a perfect life. Not only that, but everyone would also want to practice that faith so that they too could reap the benefits and rewards. It is not possible to contain the vastness of God in a human system. God is not Christian, Buddhist, Jewish, Muslim or Hindu. These are systems that were created by humans to help us to walk in and relate to the mysteries of God and help us to expand and evolve our consciousness about God.

The tendency to convince everyone to have the same religious or spiritual beliefs that I had has faded into the sunset. I no longer need to be God's defense attorney, and I can allow others to worship the God of their understanding in peace. I still have work to do on my spiritual journey by practicing the tools needed to stay peaceful and in harmony with all that is around me. But I have finally learned something comprehensive that I can consistently apply to improve my life. I feel I belong now and am a part of something bigger than myself. The stress in my life has subsided and I am more at peace. Life makes more sense and I no longer have the need to be right; I only have the need to be.

Our well-being is profoundly affected by the beliefs that we hold. It is natural for your spiritual beliefs to evolve over time, so allow yourself to go with the flow. I encourage you to evaluate your own spiritual beliefs. Dogmatic, judgmental, and unloving spiritual concepts and beliefs may manifest in our bodies as pain or illness and can have a negative effect on our ability to relate to other people.

My wish for you…

May you open your heart and be your authentic self. May you embrace ideas and beliefs that bring you ultimate wellness and peace. May you allow others the freedom to worship the God of their understanding.

On the Path - Eliminating Resistance

Man's life, in reality, is spiritual and mental, and until his thought is healed, no form of cure will be permanent.
The Science of Mind, page 190

As a young woman, I often dreamed about what it would be like to have the power to heal people. We have all seen people miraculously healed on TV, getting up out of wheelchairs and throwing away crutches. Over the years, I attended my share of healing services where the preacher had special healing powers. After he was introduced and gave his sermon, the preacher asked anyone who wanted healing to come up front. A line would form, and he would heal them one by one.

The process was almost always the same, so I pretty much knew what to expect. The preacher would inquire about the person's infirmity, then he would tell them to raise their hands and he would place his palm on their forehead. He would apply pressure to the center of their foreheads in such a way that the person would fall backwards. There was usually someone standing behind them in anticipation that they would fall to the floor, overcome by the healing power.

The preacher would say a few words or even blow on the person. Sometimes, the preacher would apply special anointing oil that was blessed in advance for the occasion.

Some would fall limp to the floor like rag dolls, while others just walked away appearing to be miraculously healed. Then there were those who were said to be "slain in the spirit" and laid out on the floor. Eventually, they would get up and stumble back to their seats, or someone would help them up.

I was a bit leery about what I saw and watched very carefully to see if people were truly healed or if they were just faking it. I remember wondering if these people were "plants" in the audience. "Were those people really healed?" I would ask myself. I wished that I could talk to them after the service to see if it was not all an act. And if the person was healed, did the healing come from the preacher or was it their belief in the preacher's ability to heal them that produced the results? How did these preachers acquire the power to heal the sick? Did they go to some kind of healer's school? I secretly prayed to be blessed with the miraculous power to heal others. With all the sickness in the world, certainly my becoming a healer was something needed.

I looked up the word "healing" in the dictionary and found that it is described as "restoring to original purity or integrity." This definition recalled to mind an old cherry handcrafted wooden bookcase that was in my office. It was the only thing I had that belonged to my grandmother and it was more than fifty years old. It was pretty beat up and I decided to restore the bookcase to see how it would turn out. I had never had any furniture restored, but for some reason, I had faith that it was possible to return the bookcase to its original state. When the restoration was complete, I was amazed at how well it turned out. The bookcase was "like new" and the memory of my grandmother was preserved. As with the bookcase, restoring our bodies to health implies that good health is already beneath the surface of any illness or disease. We only need to have faith and address the "scratches and dents" of life to align with the truth of who we are.

Some of my favorite biblical stories are the accounts of Jesus healing people, especially the story of the woman who touched the hem of his garment. This woman knew that if she could come in contact even with Jesus' clothing, she would be healed. I asked myself, "Was the healing in Jesus, or was the healing already inside of the woman?" Inasmuch as the woman knew that her healing could come from stroking a piece of clothing, I believe she simply reclaimed the healing that was already hers for the taking. Perhaps this is what Jesus meant when he said, "Daughter, your faith has healed you. Go in peace and be freed from your suffering."

There is a small wooden plaque in my bedroom with the words "Faith is the Victory" written in gold lettering. I keep it there as a reminder that Divine health is my birthright and I vibrate at a level where illness can not dwell. A friend of mine once told me that he always gets sick when the seasons change. My immediate response was, "I very rarely get sick because I do not accept sickness as my reality, and it is not part of my vocabulary. Sickness has no power over me." I have faith that I will be well, and for the most part I have been victorious.

I am blessed that I am healthy and have a high energy level. I believe that spending time each day in spiritual practices like prayer, meditation, using affirmations and visualization positively contribute to my overall wellness. I do as much as I can to keep my vibration high so that I can vibrate above the low-level energies of sickness and disease.

The Revealing Word, by Charles Filmore, offers "seekers of truth" metaphysical meanings of words and phrases that frequently appear in Unity publications and in the Bible. Filmore defines the word "healer" as one who has great compassion and yearning to help humanity out of its errors and suffering. Upon reading this, I had a profound realization that I did not need to take a course or read another book. My deep desire to help people free themselves from unhealthy lifestyles was enough. I was already the healer I yearned to become. You are also a healer and can apply the principles described in this book to your own life, or use them for your family, community, and the world around you.

If I had to use one word to describe the source of illness, it would be "resistance." Resistance is an opposing or retarding force that is created when there is imbalance or negativity. Dr. Wayne Dyer says, "Everything you are against weakens you. Everything you are for empowers you." Resistance is created when we deny what is. When we cannot change a particular circumstance, it is far better to accept it than to generate unnecessary frustration. When resistance exists, we may feel a difference in our body, like a twinge or a stress. Over time, the negative energy concentrates in a particular area of our body, blocking the natural flow of Divine wellness. This accumulation of compounded negativity creates symptoms of illness, disease, and low-level dissatisfaction.

Complaining is one way that we create resistance. The definition of the word "complain" is to express dissatisfaction, pain, uneasiness, resentment, and grief, or to find fault. For example, when we constantly complain about our pains, ailments, or hardships, we create negative energy for ourselves and for the people with whom we are sharing our complaint. We can start the healing process by becoming more aware of how often we are complaining. When we notice that we are speaking or thinking negatively about any person, place or thing, we can say "Cancel, Cancel" and change the dialogue (or monologue if we are talking to ourselves in our head) into a conversation about what we want and are grateful for. This simple exercise neutralizes the negative energy in our minds and lays the groundwork for positive changes in our circumstances.

After we neutralize the negativity, we can be thankful for the good that is within us and is reflected back to us by the universe. Appreciation, acceptance, and gratitude are three ways to bring forth the good that is within each of us. The more we focus on the good, the more it will start showing up in our life. That which we bless with gratitude multiplies and brings us more for which to be grateful.

Our relationships can bring us so much joy but at the same time bring us an equal amount of pain. There are several periods in my life when I was involved in dysfunctional romantic relationships. I believe the resistance that I carried around, especially about my relationships, was literally making me sick. No matter how hard I tried to change these situations, they only got worse. When I began to listen to my self-talk, taking inventory of how often I complained, I was astonished to discover how negative I was. I spoke pessimistically about almost everything in my life. I even had a special group of friends, and all we did was commiserate over all of the negative events in our lives.

Eventually it occurred to me that the Universe was giving me more of what I was focusing on. I decided to free myself of the painful dialogue and destructive social habits. Things changed slowly, and I soon became less disenfranchised, and the unhealthy relationships dissolved. In general, I was much more productive and spent more time thinking about how to achieve my dreams and goals. Before long, I experienced a sense of freedom and contentment.

Resistance is created when we deny reality. It is better to accept what is and make the necessary adjustments that lead toward the desired result. Now let's explore where you are on your path to ultimate wellness. Where do you go for healing? Does it come from a doctor, preacher, a potion, or a pill? Are you willing to take on the responsibility of supporting the doctor by fostering your own healing, and reclaiming your right to Divine Wellness? Is there resistance in your romantic relationships or with your family that may be obstructing healing or causing pain in your life? Are you willing to change the way you perceive, think, and talk about these areas of your life so that you can attract better health and prosperity?

My wish for you…

May you realize healing in every part of your being. May you learn to go with the flow of life. May you reclaim the rich endowment of Divine wellness.

All Roads Lead HOME (Holistic Open-Minded Evolution)

"As human beings, our greatness lies not so much in being able to remake the world…as in being able to remake ourselves."
~Mahatma Gandhi

We are taught to take care of others' needs first to avoid appearing selfish or self-centered, but the journey to wellness is our own. It is best for us to get our own act together prior to trying to help others. The Airline Safety Guidelines provide a great metaphysical lesson: In case the oxygen mask falls from the compartment above your head, put your own oxygen mask on first and then help others around you. Taking care of ourselves first allows us to be more available when we do reach out to help others. Poor self-care shows up as illness, depression, bad tempers, accidents, over-commitments, and a variety of other ways.

For us to fully address the source of a disease or debilitating life circumstance, we must restore wholeness and balance among all the dimensions of our being. When we only treat the body by giving it medicine, or only address the mind by giving it psychiatric care, we may be neglecting other aspects of our being that also need care. When we begin to recognize areas that have been neglected, we can use specific practices to treat the area in need of attention and promote overall wellness.

In the James Allen classic that was transcribed for women by Dorothy J. Hulst entitled *As A Woman Thinketh*, the following quote reveals the need to harmonize our inner and outer worlds.

> "A woman is not rightly conditioned until she is a happy, healthy, and prosperous being and happiness, health, and prosperity are the result of a harmonious adjustment of the inner with the outer, of the woman with her surroundings."

My interpretation of the "inner" and the "outer" that Allen is referring to is the relationship between the visible and the invisible aspects of our being, namely our mind, body, and soul with our surrounding space. I refer to this multi-dimensional existence as the "Holistic Matrix."

Holistic Matrix

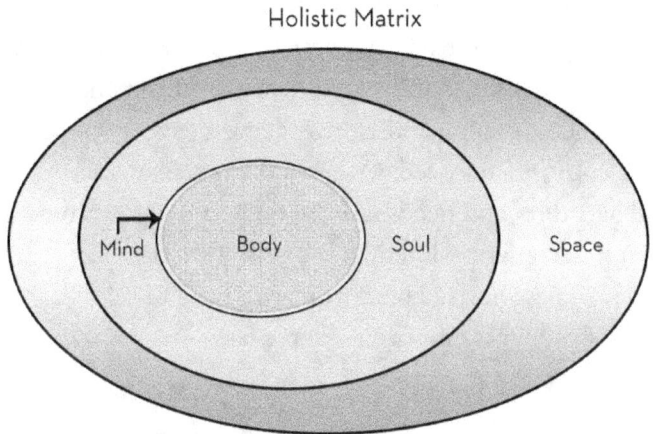

As illustrated in the above diagram, the mind fully engulfs our body, and our body is enveloped by the soul. Since everything is energy, our mind, body, and soul influence the space that surrounds us; and our environment has a reciprocal impact on us as well. Below is a brief description of each part of the Holistic Matrix.

The Mind

Science supports the idea that our attitudes and emotions have an influence on the functioning of the body, and that most, if not all, disease is psychosomatic in origin. When we speak about the mind, we are usually referring to the aspects of intellect and consciousness manifested as combinations of thought, memory, and emotion. The mind is not the same thing as the brain. The brain is the organ encased by our skull, but the mind is the consciousness that exists in every cell of our body, which is how we make our body parts move on command. The mind is like a car transmission; it keeps the body running at the appropriate speed. Over time, the transmission fluid gets dirty and needs a flush. So, it is with our mind when it becomes polluted with negative thoughts of perceived past hurts. This is when we need to release and let go of thoughts that do not serve us.

The Body

Every day, we see images of perfect bodies that we will never have, and many people struggle in some way with their physical inadequacies. Our culture has convinced us that our bodies are who we are. Dr. Björn Nordenström, a Swedish radiologist, did twelve years of research on the nature of the physical body as an energetic phenomenon. His findings concluded that the body is associated with an energy field that exists within and around the body, but it is not produced by the body. The energy field that makes the body is the mind, and our thoughts and feelings influence the energy field. Dr. Nordenström demonstrated that a chemical or physical abnormality in the body is caused by a disturbance in the energy field that produces the body.

Our body can give us clues when something is out of synch. Learning to listen to the messages that our body is telling us is critical to achieving ultimate wellness. An analogy to help to describe this concept is the tire pressure light on the dashboard of my car. Not long after I purchased the car, a light came on to indicate that there was a problem with my tires, but I drove around for a month before I made the time to bring the car into the dealership. When my car was inspected, they found a nail in the rear tire that could have potentially caused me serious harm if it had continued to go unattended. Stress and tension are our body's sensors that let us know when we are out of balance. The key to a healthy lifestyle is to pay attention to the sensors and take care of our body's needs before things get too serious.

The Soul

The soul exists separately from the body and consists of our consciousness and personality. Ernest Holmes wrote about the soul as being a mirror of the mind reflecting the forms of thought. *The Revealing Word* states that our bodily health reflects the state of the soul. Our thoughts affect the way we feel, and our feelings are the language of the soul and influence the energy field that makes the body. We can consciously feed the soul with good thoughts and expect that optimal circumstances will be the result.

An analogy for how the soul works is the accelerator and the brake pedals in our car. When we think negative thoughts, it is like we are intermittently stomping on the brake pedal, which creates a bumpy and uncomfortable ride in life. When we think positive thoughts, we are pressing the accelerator, which allows things to go more smoothly and with the flow of life.

Our Space

We often overlook the environments that surround and unavoidably impact our lives. Our homes can be viewed as our outer body and can provide clues as to what is going on with our health, particularly when there is a problem. Our living space is like the body of a car. Although there might be a few nicks and dents on the surface, it protects the motor that keeps the car operating. But if there is serious damage to the body, it impacts how the car functions. The same is true for our living space. Negative energy or unsupportive living conditions disturb the balance of our mind, body, and soul, which promotes disease.

Beating the Wicked Witch of the West

My favorite movie of all time is *The Wizard of Oz*, directed by Victor Fleming. In it, Dorothy dreams of a better place, "somewhere over the rainbow." After being struck unconscious during a tornado, she dreams that she is transported from Kansas to the magical Land of Oz. Dorothy's inner and outer worlds are connected, as Oz contains reflections of the characters and events of her life in Kansas. Throughout the movie, her only goal is to return home to Kansas. On her journey down the Yellow Brick Road, Dorothy must find her own way. As she advances towards the Emerald City, she encounters many strange and frightening occurrences. Glenda, the Good Witch of the North, provides Dorothy with guidance but allows her to make her own discoveries.

During Dorothy's journey to Oz, she meets the Scarecrow, the Tin Man, and the Cowardly Lion, who join her, hoping to receive what they themselves lack (a brain, a heart and courage, respectively). These characters could reflect parts of Dorothy's being that need treatment. For example, the Scarecrow represents the mind, the Tin Man, the soul, the Cowardly Lion, the body, and the Yellow Brick Road represents her space. To find her way home, Dorothy must integrate all of the parts of her being and overcome a number of challenges while also trying to avoid the Wicked Witch of the West (illness and repeated patterns of negative circumstances) who threatens her life.

Like Dorothy, I had my struggles and personal afflictions. If it was not a failed marriage or relationship, it was my job or a financial issue. The names and faces changed, but the core issues remained the same. I was telling the same old stories repeatedly, like a broken record. My life was continuously plagued by strikingly similar circumstances that put me in a bad mood. I read every self-help and spiritual book I could get my hands on and I came to one important conclusion: I am the common denominator for everything that shows up in my life. I soon realized that to overcome my personal Wicked Witch of the West, I had to let go of trying to fix other people; stop trying to fix the circumstances outside of me and navigate my own way to ultimate wellness.

There are many roads to healing from an internal perspective as well as on the physical plane. If we look at how well we are meeting our own needs, we often find that we have been neglecting our own care. There are several tools in Part Two of this book to help us to make subtle adjustments to the mind, body, soul, or space so that we can live happier, more fulfilling lives.

Anything that disturbs the balance of our mind, body, soul, or our relationship with our environment promotes disease. I am wondering if you reach out to help others before you address your own needs. Do you feel that you are worthy enough to give yourself time each day? Are you listening to the messages that your body is sending you? Does your treatment of illness or imbalance address all aspects of your Being?

My wish for you…

May you learn to take better care of yourself. May you pay attention to your body's signals. May you only think thoughts that foster vitality and wellness. May your Yellow Brick Road lead you to a more Holistic, Open-Minded Evolution (HOME).

The Journey Inwards

"The longest journey is the journey inwards."
~ Dag Hammarskjøld

It has become increasingly clear to me that how we react to life circumstances is driven by what is going on inside of us. I consider myself to be a spiritual person and practice spiritual principles so that I can maintain the highest level of peace and harmony around me. When everything is status quo, I do quite well, and I live a fulfilled life. Most of the time, I try to resolve issues with a cool head, but when my back is up against the wall, it can sometimes be quite different.

I began to question why whenever there is a problem or disagreement it is a little more difficult to respond in loving ways. I found the answer in a book called, *In the Flow of Life* by Eric Butterworth. In his book, Butterworth tells a story about a woman who was upset because someone had taken her seat on the train. She was very disturbed about it and called the person "an animal." Butterworth explains,

> It is a difficult lesson, but an important one, to admit that your sudden flare-up of anger evidenced that beneath the façade of composure, there was chaos within you that morning. Thus, you were disturbed by what happened because you were disturbable. If you

had been in a more loving consciousness, you probably would have dealt with the whole thing in an entirely different way.

When the "little me" surfaces, it's an indication that I am "disturbable," which actually attracts events and situations that cause me to express the suppressed feelings within. Instead, I should take a deeper look at myself to determine the underlying cause of my dissatisfaction. While traveling on the interstate, I noticed a Jim Beam bourbon advertisement on the side of a truck that caught my eye: "The stuff inside matters most." It is such a simple point, but it speaks volumes and is true on so many levels. Our attitude, the way that we treat people, the situations and circumstances going on in our lives are merely reflections of what is going on inside.

One of the things that could be causing inner dissatisfaction is when our basic needs are not being met. During my college days, I learned about Abraham Maslow, an American psychologist noted for his conceptualization of a "hierarchy of human needs." According to Maslow, we are motivated by our unsatisfied needs as we seek to realize our greatest potential. With his model, our lower physiological needs (breathing, food, water, sex, sleep, and excretion) and safety needs (security of body, employment, resources, morality, family, and health) must be satisfied before the need to be loved and to belong (friendship, family and intimacy) emerges. The theory is that we must satisfy these lower needs before we can develop our highest sense of self (self-esteem, confidence, and achievement).

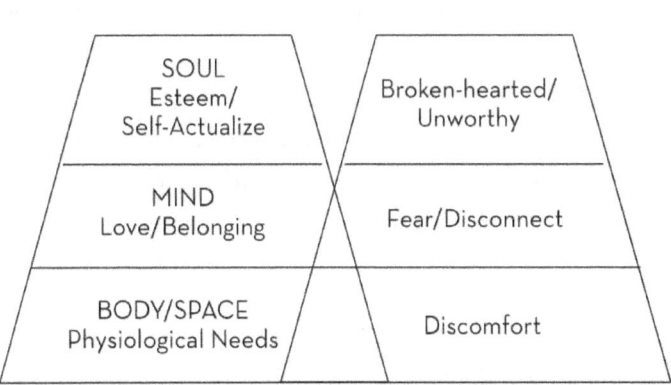

Holistic Hierarchy

Taking Maslow's building-block-based theory a step further, we can correlate Maslow's levels of need with the different facets of our being: mind, body, soul, and space, in what I call the Holistic Hierarchy. We are motivated to rise up the hierarchy as we address the root cause of our problems. For example, at the lowest level, we want to live in a safe place, and be comfortable in our bodies and our space.

A friend shared with me that she was unable to get her own place and had to live with a family member. No matter what she did, she could not get comfortable there and was very unhappy. My friend's discomfort was creating resistance by making her resentful about not having her own place. If she failed to resolve the way that she saw her current space, she could very possibly recreate the same condition even after she found a new home. This resistance showed up in her body as stress in her lower back and headaches. Left unattended, these symptoms could have developed into a full-blown disease. The build-up of resistance also created negative energy in her space. Anyone who entered the space could sense that the tension in the air was thick enough to cut with a knife.

Dr. Wayne Dyer said, "If you change the way that you look at things, the things you look at change." One way my friend began to resolve her issue was to make peace with the space that was available to her and to be grateful that she was not living on the street. I shared this Maya Angelou quote with her, "I long, as does every human being, to be at home wherever I find myself." When my friend began to act like a person who was "at home" by taking care of the space that was provided for her, she felt more welcomed and at home.

From a health perspective, we can accept our current state as it is by showing gratitude for the health that we do have. Then we could begin doing the things that healthy people do, by taking care of our bodies and ensuring that we have a healthy regimen of eating well and exercising. When we live as though we are already healthy, the way we perceive our health will change.

Once we are comfortable and safe, we progress to the next level of the Holistic Hierarchy, which is "Love and Belonging." It has been said that there are only two emotions: love and fear. If we are not coming from a place of love, then we are living in fear. Fear is an acronym for "False Evidence Appearing Real" and is often created out of a false pretense or negative thinking. This fear creates resistance, which could open a portal for ill health to set in. When we think that we are all alone or get lonely, we can feel disconnected from the world around us. Accepting the idea that we are all one and part of the One Mind allows us to feel more connected to God, to people and to everything we see and touch. This thought helps us to "plug" ourselves back in to the "socket" of life.

When we are comfortable and able to accept the love that is all around us, we progress to the highest level of the hierarchy. At the pinnacle level, we begin to evaluate our self-worth and the contribution that we want to make to the world. We may start asking questions like: "Who am I?" and "Why am I here?" We have all suffered from some degree of feeling unworthy and became emotionally distraught. If we are hurting, suffering from an illness, or having difficulty forgiving someone, it's usually because we are holding on to pain from the past. We can elevate our consciousness by learning to love ourselves more. When we become the love that we are seeking, feelings of unworthiness and past pain fade away.

This foundational evolutionary model allows us to resolve the core issues of discomfort, fear and unworthiness within us and embark on the inward journey toward optimal healing and ultimate wellness. Utilizing a holistic approach allows us to address the root cause of our issues, which helps us to avoid perpetuating similar situations in the future.

Whatever we focus on expands. When we think as though we are already living the life we want, more of it will manifest for us. I am interested to know if discomfort shows up for you in your body or home. And what about your fears? Can you also feel them in your body? Do you ever experience loneliness or feel like you are all alone? Do you feel worthy enough to be loved by others?

My wish for you...

May you be more in tune with what is going on in your inner realm. May you find comfort in your total being. May you be that which you are seeking and attract it into your life.

Who Are You Being?

"Happiness is not a matter of intensity but of balance, order, rhythm and harmony." ~ Thomas Merton

In the last chapter, I shared how fully resolving our unmet needs can help to promote healing and achieve ultimate wellness. Now we will shift our focus to ways that we may attain greater balance among the different dimensions of our being. Learning to balance our mind, body, and soul with the space that surrounds us is crucial to achieving greater wellness. When we operate predominately from our intellect, the other aspects of our being may be out of balance. The same holds true when our body is of primary importance, our spirituality is overbearing, or we make the space we live in more important than anything else. The four character traits below help us to look at who we are being and offer ways to resolve any disparity.

Magnified Mind

We magnify our mind when we are predominately focused on intellect. Education is wonderful, but you are more than your education. There were times in my life when I felt I needed to learn more before I could write a book, accept a speaking engagement or share my personal views. I felt that I needed just one more class, seminar, or degree. If I waited until I had everything that I thought was required, I could have potentially died with my dreams still in me.

When we operate predominately from the mind, we risk being ruled by the ego. You may demonstrate this behavior when you stick to old opinions and beliefs and defend them at all costs to keep from being wrong. It may even show up when you act like you know all the answers, even to things you know nothing about. There may even be times when you over-think a situation so much that you do not listen to your inner guide. We all exhibit these behaviors but when they are in excess, it may be a sign that you are magnifying your mind.

Bill Gates, a major philanthropist and one of the wealthiest men alive, has helped millions of people through his vision to computerize the world. I have learned a valuable lesson from this Harvard dropout: When I am authentic and share from my heart, I touch lives in positive ways.

When we magnify our mind, it diminishes our ability to live fully balanced lives, and we may be less in tune with our intuition (soul) and out of touch with what is going on around us (space). We may neglect the needs of our body due to the importance placed on the intellect. Living a life primarily through the mind could also make us robotic, lifeless, and mechanical.

Body Booster

A Body Booster type operates from a body-dominated perspective. Body Boosters focus excessively on their bodies and may be fixated on satisfying the desires of the flesh. These people may also live to eat rather than eat to live, or they may deprive themselves of food so that they can maintain a certain weight. Body Boosters may not see the value in spirituality (soul) and may not be interested in what is going on around them (space). These people may prefer to spend time in the gym more than reading books or having an intellectual conversation (mind).

I remember the days when I was preoccupied with my body. I never thought that I was beautiful and wore lots of make-up and revealing clothing to get attention. I felt that I needed to be a certain dress size to be accepted and attractive. Now I am more interested in comfortable clothing and maintaining a healthy regimen rather than being obsessed with the size of my body.

Operating predominately from the body could cause you to be dependent on your looks, which could create a problem, especially as you begin to age. When the body no longer appears youthful, this could result in a loss of self-esteem. To achieve more balance, Body Boosters could try to get in touch with what is inside their beautiful bodies by asking probing questions like, "What would bring more value into my life and the world?" Answering these types of questions may help to create a greater balance with their soul, mind, and space.

Sinfully Soulful

There was a time that I thought that living purely from my soul would bring me happiness, but I soon discovered that this lifestyle also created an imbalance. I met a genuinely nice lady from church who talked about God all the time. I do not know exactly what was wrong with her, but she was overweight and walked very slowly with a cane. She was married and had two toddlers and a terribly busy schedule. Not only that, but she was also in church almost every night of the week. I had reason to visit her home to work with her on a project. What I saw shocked me. Her home, while it looked good on the outside, was in shambles on the inside. There were things everywhere covering the floor and countertops. It was difficult for me to concentrate because I was distracted by all the stuff that seemed to be closing in on me.

Operating mainly from the soul may appear to be the preferred path, but this behavior also causes an imbalance. Being Sinfully Soulful created an imbalance in my friend's life and resulted in an unhealthy lifestyle for her and her family. If she were to learn to pay more attention to the other aspects of her being, this would bring about greater balance with her mind, body and space.

Superior Space

Superior Space types place a great value on how things look on the outside and give less attention to their mind, body, or soul. People preoccupied with space may have a propensity to be materialistic and be driven by acquiring new things. This type may seek to have all the latest gadgets before they come on the market, and they will be prepared to stand in long lines to experience the privileges of ownership. They may also continue shopping even after their money runs out and there is no room left in their closets.

Superior Space types may also suffer from "Retail Therapy," the psychological condition where people shop for the primary purpose of improving their mood or disposition because the sensation of shopping makes them feel better. When Superior Space types become more conscious of the other aspects of themselves, their desire to gain more "stuff" will diminish. In addition, addressing the underlying imbalance will help to resolve debt issues associated with the shopping habit.

On a chilly winter night as I was leaving an engagement, I noticed several guys sitting in lawn chairs outside a commercial establishment. It looked rather odd, as they wrapped themselves in blankets, and I couldn't help but ask what they were doing. One gentleman proudly responded that a new pair of tennis shoes was going to be available the next morning and they were going to sleep there overnight to ensure that they got a pair. At the risk of catching pneumonia, these Superior Space character types maintained the need for material possessions over the need to care for their bodies.

We all exhibit a combination of the above traits at varying levels. However, when one trait is predominant, it could have a negative impact on our health and life circumstances. Consider taking the time to examine when the traits above are out of balance. When we let go of old ideas that no longer serve us and release the need to be right, we can create a space for more balance to flow through our soul, body, and space. Once we become more aware of whom we are being, then we can begin to bring our total being into balance and live more fulfilled lives.

Becoming more conscious of who we are being allows us to make the adjustments necessary to live a healthier life. I am curious if your personality is aligned with the Magnified Mind, Body Booster, Sinfully Soulful or the Superior Space character traits. In what areas of your life do you see the imbalance showing up the most? How can you realign yourself so that you are more balanced?

My wish for you...

May you be more aware of when you are operating in imbalanced ways. May you learn how to restore the joy to your life. May you find balance in your mind, body, soul and your space to achieve ultimate wellness.

The Corridor of Cause

"To make a deep physical path, we walk again and again. To make a deep mental path, we must think over and over the kind of thoughts we wish to dominate our lives." ~ Henry David Thoreau

I once worked at one of the best jobs that I have ever had in my entire working career. I enjoyed it because I had a great deal of flexibility and no one was breathing down my neck. I liked helping people to solve their problems, but I had far too many clients than I could feasibly serve. Some of them were rude and felt that having their desires met superseded any need to be courteous towards me. Many times, I allowed them to disrespect me because I was fearful that I would lose my job. If I lost my job, then I would not be able to pay my bills. If I could not pay my bills… Well, you know the rest of the story.

I was also exhibiting fear in other areas of my life. For example, I bent over backwards to please my mate because I was fearful that he would not want me if I did not do things for him. I loved to sing but was afraid that people would not like my voice. I experienced tremendous fear whenever I would get up in front of others to speak for fear that I would make a mistake or forget what I wanted to say and people would laugh at me. I always wanted to write a book but was fearful to express my ideas and views because they were different from the norm.

The list goes on and on. It is sad to say, but I was living in a constant state of fear. I could feel the fear in different parts of my body. Most of the time I could feel it in my chest area; other times I felt the fear in my throat or abdominal area. Then there were times when I could feel it in my wrists, back, legs and feet. The fear was blocking the natural flow of energy in my body and my life.

My depressing circumstances stemmed from holding on to resentment and unfinished business from the past. The serious emotional traumas that I experienced negatively affected my state of mind. My internal conflicts were on an unconscious level and I was not aware of them. I was broken-hearted and had feelings of shame and guilt. Many of my problems relating to my health, marriage, business, employment, and children had connections rooted in the fear I subconsciously held in my mind. Thinking and talking negatively about my situation only gave it more power and recreated similar circumstances in my future. Getting another job, a new boyfriend or new friends only gave me momentary relief.

Emmett Fox provides insight on how to resolve the root cause of our issues: "

> If people are troublesome, you have only to change your thought about them, and then they will change too, because your own concept is what you see.

I had to take a good look at myself and make the necessary shifts in my thought processes, which changed my viewpoint and gave me a new perspective.

In 2006, a friend shared an extremely popular DVD with me called *The Secret* by Rhonda Byrne, which touted the "Law of Attraction" as the most powerful law of the universe. This movie helped me to understand that we attract every circumstance into our life with our thoughts and we are using this principle whether we are aware of it or not. We have the choice to attract good or bad situations into our lives all the time. Once we better understand how the process works, we can consciously manifest what we really want into our lives. Our thoughts vibrate out at a positive or negative frequency. They manifest outwardly and draw that which is of a similar frequency like a magnet. The idea comes first, and then the structure to support it. It is thought that sets the creative wheels in motion outwards and then displays what was once hidden inside of the mind.

My mantra is "I Create My Own Reality." What this means is that I am responsible for whatever is showing up in my life. Taking full responsibility for the content of my thoughts unleashes my power to change any situation that is unacceptable to me. If I continue to blame others, then I must depend on them to fix my problems.

Taking responsibility for our circumstances rather than feeling victimized or blaming others is a significant first step in addressing them. If we get sick, have an accident or run into tough times, we're likely to protest that we did not have these kinds of thoughts and ask, "How could I be responsible?" The probable cause is likely rooted in events that have long been forgotten.

For example, a woman's terminal illness gets her the attention she lacked as a little girl. An artist's career ends when he embraces the restrictive beliefs of a religious cult that offers the structure he missed in childhood. In both cases, the true cause of the problem was unconscious, though the person probably would have vigorously denied its existence. The hidden cause brought about consequences that corresponded to it. Once we take responsibility for our circumstances, we can look at our problems as a reflection of hidden aspects of ourselves and begin the healing process.

In my former days as a computer programmer there was a saying, garbage in–garbage out. That meant that the computer program can only do what it is instructed to do. Likewise, we frequently program ourselves with words and thoughts that are not healthy. Every word that you utter and every thought that you think, has a vibration, and sets energy into motion. Much like a genie in a bottle, the Universe replicates the vibration and manifests your words and thoughts into form. If everything is working for you, then keep doing what you are doing. But if you want a different output, you must change the input. Like a computer program, garbage in equates to garbage out.

Things that we say every day that are part of our normal vocabulary could be hurting our health and chances for success. Do you ever use phrases like the ones below?

"You kill me…"

"That really blew my mind…"

"I almost died when…"

"It hit me like a ton of bricks…"

"I was floored…"

"You make me sick…"

"Give me a break…"

"You crack me up…"

"You are a pain in the neck…"

"It struck me that…"

"I'm dying to see you…"

"I'm going to blow up!"

These slang terms can be far from innocent and may bring harmful results if used regularly. One of my mother's favorite lines is, "It's always something," meaning that there is always some problem that she is faced with. Oddly enough, she is frequently involved in some kind of drama with the people around her. The Universe always delivers her "something" on a silver platter because she speaks it into existence.

Our thoughts and words are immensely powerful and do manifest into form good or bad. A guy I know likes to use the slang expression "it hit me in the head," meaning that an idea or concept became clear to him. When I met him he was in the middle of a Workers Compensation case because he was hurt on the job. He showed me the heavy corroded metal lamppost cap that fell twenty feet, knocking him unconscious and putting a deep gash in his head. He may not want to admit it but there is a high probability that his words were manifested into reality. Confirmation of this came about a year later when he contacted me with excitement in his voice. He showed me the book that I gave him during our life-coaching sessions. One of the exercises was to create a Vision for his life which required that he write down what he wanted in every area of his life. He was ecstatic when he told me that everything that he wrote down had manifested, including getting a major record deal with a well-known artist, which pays him handsome royalties.

On every level, we are creating what is showing up in our lives; however, it appears that much of what we are thinking is unconscious. Every condition is in accordance with the unfailing law of causation. I have grown very conscious of the "power of the tongue," and the power of my thoughts. I am incredibly careful with the words I use and very cautious about saying anything that I do not wish to come to fruition. We have the creative power to shape our lives according to our own mental patterns. The things we manifest are the direct effects of the thoughts hidden in our minds and the words that flow out of our mouth.

I do not believe that anyone gets sick or attracts harm on purpose, but I do believe that we are responsible for creating the particular corner of the world that we experience each day. Letting go of all the perceived notions of the past and reawakening to a new you is a major part of achieving ultimate wellness. The key is to learn to release those things that no longer serve you and embrace ideas that serve and support you. You can do this by paying closer attention to the thoughts that continuously flow through your head, then gently guiding your thoughts from fear to the things that you genuinely want. Take note of what you have been choosing, and if it is not producing the desired effect, then choose again.

If we want to improve our lives, it requires that we begin to shift our mental focus from the problem to the solution. This allows us to release limiting thoughts and to achieve the breakthrough that we seek. Take time to turn your thoughts from moods of insufficiency to attitudes of confidence, from thoughts of lack and limitation to prosperity and abundance, from thoughts of sickness to thoughts of ultimate health.

The process of healing requires that we begin to shift our mental focus from the problem to the solution. I'm wondering about you now. Do you also have fears that you have lived with all your life? How have those fears stunted your growth? And what about your language? Do you use words that are harmful to your well-being?

My wish for you…

May the meditations of your heart reveal that which you truly desire. May your words be true, kind, necessary and healing. May you be guided from pain to peace, from fear to love and from hell to heaven.

Now Is the Time

"Do not dwell in the past; do not dream of the future; concentrate the mind on the present moment." ~ *Buddha*

I was heading to a facial appointment one Saturday morning and took my normal route through town. I had only gone a mile or so before I noticed that the traffic had come to a complete standstill. This was very unusual as I had traveled this road for many years and never experienced any type of delay.

Upon closer evaluation of the situation, I noticed that there were orange cones blocking off the street, and the police were ahead. It appeared that there was some type of group walking for a cause, because I caught a glimpse of the people passing by. I had not heard about any special event, but it became clear to me that the delay would be a while. I had given myself plenty of time, so I did not panic or get upset. There was not anything I could do but wait.

The gentleman in the car directly behind me caught my attention when he started blowing his horn. I watched him through my rear-view mirror as he got visibly upset and started banging his hand on the steering wheel. In a matter of minutes, he stepped out of his car and began shouting. Then he got back into his car and started shaking his hands frantically in quick motions, then banging his hand against the passenger seat. My concern was elevated as he tried to maneuver his way out of the jam, because there was nowhere that he could go. This went on for about five minutes until the traffic opened. I thanked God that things ended without incident.

As the gentleman passed me, I wondered if this was his typical behavior. I contemplated what it must be like to live or work with a person who was unable to tolerate a six-minute traffic jam. This incident reminded me of other people in my life who were rude, disrespectful, and impatient. Then I turned my focus to myself and recalled the many times that I too failed to exhibit patience.

The man in the car behind me created a lot of resistance and negative energy in that moment, but I chose to remain calm. Patience is a choice, and I learned to be more patient because I know that impatience only creates resistance to what is. This resistance not only lodges itself in the body, but also pollutes the entire universe. Our health is influenced by our attitudes and emotions. Resistance begins in the mind and self-limiting attitudes inhibit the natural flow of life. Financial worries, poor work conditions, emotional upsets, fear of losing a job, et cetera, all dam up the naturally good flow of energy inside of you. The cells of the body take their cue from our mental state and cause blockage and congestion. These conditions impede our natural flow but can be easily adjusted by learning to live in the present moment.

Eckhart Tolle is an expert on staying in the present moment. In his book, *The Power of Now*, Tolle teaches about becoming aware of the space of now. "You suddenly feel more alive inside. You feel the aliveness of the inner body – the aliveness that is an intrinsic part of the joy of Being." One way that we can live in the now is by staying conscious of what we are thinking and feeling. If you are feeling anxiousness or nervousness in your body, you may be thinking too much about the future. If you are feeling down or depressed, you may be spending too much time lamenting over the past. Let's take a closer look at how too much past or too much future can negatively impact our lives.

Too Much Past

"So many people miss their blessings because they are still lamenting unhappy experiences of the past." ~ Catherine Ponder

I met a gentleman who was a great conversationalist, and I enjoyed hearing his stories about his grandmother and great-grandmother. As time went on, I noticed that he had an unusually keen memory of his grade school friends, and all his teachers' names. I thought that this was an extraordinary gift. He talked a lot about the old days, his old friends, and the time that he spent in the military twenty years earlier. He also vividly relived the negative aspects of his failed marriage and talked about his divorce in excruciating detail. As we got closer, I discovered things that seemed peculiar. There was a life-sized baby doll and a miniature rocking chair in his den that belonged to his estranged teenage daughter whom he had not seen since she was a little girl. I thought nothing of it, and just felt that maybe he was a little sentimental.

Then I noticed other things that caused me concern. Although I do not have the greatest sense of smell, I noticed that his twenty-year-old oversized outdated furniture smelled like mildew. Many of the clothes in his closet were incredibly old and no longer fit him. There were boxes of old clothes and uniforms in his spare bedroom closet that had dry-rotted, but he refused to part with them. His car was twelve years old, and he invested twelve thousand dollars in it in a matter of months so that he could continue to drive it. He had a large collection of VHS videotapes of old movies and hundreds of cassette tapes that were major dust-collectors. Daily, he spent countless hours watching old syndicated black-and-white movies. I think that you are starting to get the picture.

In isolation, any one of these scenarios does not seem to be an issue. But when you look at the total picture, it could indicate that this guy was more comfortable with his past than he was with the present or future. This was coupled with the fact that he was verbally and physically abusive towards people and had major problems with his mother and his daughters. Moreover, he was overweight and suffered from diabetes, high cholesterol, and high blood pressure.

When we live in the past, we are oblivious to the present and future. Reliving past pain creates negative feelings such as anger, resentment, jealousy, and guilt. Holding grudges or beating yourself up about something you did that caused someone pain, suffering or harm could be a sign that you are creating too much past.

Spending lots of time talking and thinking about the past could be another indication that we are creating too much past, which could be harmful to our health. If there are people you have not forgiven for something they did to you in the past or you intentionally hurt another person, this could reveal that you are living in the past. There is an old saying: "A fool loses tomorrow looking back at yesterday." There is not anything that you can do about the past, except let it go and move on. Get in touch with how you are feeling and use this as a reminder to shift towards living in the present.

Too Much Future

I used to wake up each morning with a feeling of anxiety about the different aspects of my life. I also felt this way whenever I had a morning appointment, because I was nervous that I would oversleep. Day after day, I had noticed my posture was future-oriented, as I would catch myself leaning forward in my office chair or in my car as I raced to get somewhere or finish something. For years, it was standard practice for me to set the clock in my car at least ten minutes ahead because I did not ever want to be late.

At times when I was super-busy, I would get very anxious, because I was thinking about how much I had to do with the limited time that was available to me. From time to time, I would even have trouble catching my breath and my chest felt tight. These were physiological signs that I was spending too much time thinking about the future and was out of touch with the present. As a result, I was always preoccupied with something on my mind, and not fully present in the company of others. There were also times when I was impatient and cut people off when they were talking to me.

We live in a microwave society where everyone wants everything now. We pack our days with activities and are in a constant rush to get where we are going. To help me to stay in the present moment, I limit my activities and I have learned how to say no. I like the way that Pema Chodron put it when she said, "Now is the only time. How we relate to it creates the future." Slowing myself down is no longer an option, but an integral part of my routine. Now I spend more time smelling the roses of life and doing things that I enjoy. As I go about my day, I remember to take deep breaths when I am feeling a little flustered. I find that listening to soft music helps keep me calm and reduce my anxiety.

Living in the present moment requires that we continuously look inward to observe our emotions and our physiological reactions. You can determine if you are living in the past or focusing too much on the future by getting in touch with how you are feeling. If you find that you are not in the moment, take a few deep breaths and remind yourself that now is the only time that we have for sure.

What about you, dear reader? Can you identify more with the past than you can with what is going on in your life right now? Are you living fully in the present moment? Do you find yourself spending a great deal of time thinking about the past or the future?

My wish for you…

May you be free from stress and strain. May you go forward in life unhurried and unworried. May you release the past that no longer serves you. May you find healing and comfort in this very moment.

PART TWO

A Holistic Approach to Wellness

"The...patient should be made to understand that he or she must take charge of his own life. Don't take your body to the doctor as if he were a repair shop." ~ Quentin Regestein

There are hundreds of ways to approach wholeness and vitality, but many require that you break through traditional beliefs, theories, perspectives, and methods. Treating the symptoms only, may not eliminate the root cause of most chronic illnesses or psychological conditions. The increased use of both traditional and alternative medicine combined has proven to be more effective than using these methods independently.

In the words of Albert Einstein, "In the middle of every difficulty lies opportunity." Whether we are dealing with ill health or a life crisis, we can participate in our healing. I have been told by people who have experienced life-threatening illnesses that they believe the illness came as a teacher to show them that they needed to slow down and take better care of themselves.

In the prior chapters, we looked at how the various dimensions of our being can get out of balance. On the pages that follow are several time-tested methods to heal the mind, body, soul, and space that can be easily applied for busy lifestyles. Since one person's journey to wellness may not work for another, there are several practices offered in each section. Choose the practice that resonates with you the most, and let your soul be your guide.

Mind Therapy

"Your health is the sum total of all the impulses, positive and negative, emanating from your consciousness. You are what you think." ~ Deepak Chopra

There is incredible healing power and intelligence within you. Healing takes many forms and does not always show up as the curing of a physical ailment. Healing may manifest as peace of mind about a challenging situation, the ability to deal with a difficult relationship, renewed inner strength or letting go of old anger. You can heal your mind by changing negative and limiting thoughts to thoughts that are positive and uplifting.

You can open yourself up to more positive experiences through practices like forgiveness, affirmations, and visualizations. Forgiveness releases us from the perceived mistakes and failures of the past. Affirmations help us retrain the mind to focus on and attract what we genuinely want. Visualizations allow us to use the power of imagination to communicate with our brain through pictures. When we learn how to use these practices, we can activate our own indwelling healing potential.

Forgiveness Freeway

"We must develop and maintain the capacity to forgive. He who is devoid of the power to forgive is devoid of the power to love. There is some good in the worst of us and some evil in the best of us." ~Martin Luther King, Jr.

Early in my career, I worked for a Fortune 500 company for almost fourteen years, but I felt like a misfit. I did not particularly enjoy the work, and it seemed like my bosses were always on my case. The people were nice, but for the most part, there was a lot of office politics and gossiping. I was a single parent at the time and did not feel like I had any other options, so I had to grin and bear it.

One morning on a typical workday, I ventured off to work. As I listened to the radio, I noticed something in the sky. I could not make out what it was, but it appeared to be getting larger and larger. As I traveled down the highway, I noticed that the object was quickly growing in mid-air. It occurred to me that the object was growing because it was getting closer to me. In a matter of seconds, I realized that the object was a tractor-trailer-sized tire heading full throttle towards my car.

I was horrified and did not know whether to slow down or speed up. The large piece of black rubber probably weighed a hundred pounds and seemed to be traveling faster than the speed of light. I said a quick prayer and, in that moment, I decided that no harm would come to my vehicle or me. Thankfully, the tire just missed my car, and I was able to get to work without incident. After this experience, I realized that it was time for me to make another choice about my job.

I decided to find work where I did not have to travel along the beltway but did not address the built-up resentment towards having to go to work each day. About ten years later, I had another opportunity to learn how negative thoughts and behavior bring about more undesirable experiences. I was experiencing similar circumstances with another job that I did not enjoy. Day in and day out I complained about one thing or another that disappointed me. One day while driving to a meeting for work I noticed a brick ricocheting along the highway. In seconds the brick surfaced from underneath the car in front of me and skidded across the hood of my car, leaving several deep gashes. I thanked God that it was not worse, yet it was another reminder to reverse my long-term negativity.

Extended periods of painful unhappiness can negatively impact our health and cause serious illness. Dr. Frederic Luskin conducted the Stanford Forgiveness Project, which validated that the practice of forgiveness has been proven to reduce anger, hurt depression and stress, and leads to greater feelings of hope, peace, compassion and self confidence. Practicing forgiveness not only leads to healthier relationships it also improves physical health.

In her book, *You Can Heal Your Life,* Louise Hay describes cancer as "deep hurt," "longstanding resentment," "deep secret or grief eating away at the self" and "carrying hatreds." I realized my resentments towards my employers were like a cancer. Knowing this alarmed me and I vowed to resolve the root cause before I had an even bigger problem on my hands.

The practice of forgiveness is a means of freeing ourselves from the bondage of resentment. Forgiveness frees us from the pain of blaming others, releases the need to be a victim and allows room for the possibility of error or weakness in ourselves and others. There are no perfect people or situations. When we forgive, it brings our thoughts into alignment with all of the good of the Universe. Forgiving others and our self releases the past and heals our heart.

Forgiveness work is a continuous process and should be repeated often. I did not create the resentment towards my employers overnight, and I gave myself time to work it through. I chose to forgive myself for viewing my employers negatively and forgave them for how I perceived they treated me. While doing forgiveness work, I find it useful to also send loving energy towards those whom I felt had done me an injustice. This act helps to unclog any blockages and allows good energy to flow. Once I had fully forgiven my employer, I found that I had an easier time at work.

Forgiving Yourself

Life is about learning to live consciously and honoring who we are in the moment. We make many choices in our lifetime. Some choices we are proud of, while others make us wish we had made better decisions. Forgiveness is a personal tool that can be used to help us heal from past mistakes or beliefs. It helps us to be gentler with ourselves as we navigate through life. When we choose to think something negative, forgiveness is most likely necessary. If we perceive anything other than love, goodness and grace within ourselves or toward others, we must free ourselves from judgment. Forgiveness is a way that we can change our old patterns, beliefs and actions that stem from unresolved issues and bitterness.

Forgiveness of Others

Sometimes the things we think are hurtful were never intended to be. Refuse to harbor negative feelings toward anyone or carry the sorrows and mistakes of the past. When we hold resentment against anyone, we are bound to him or her. When we hold on to anger and pain, we can make ourselves sick. Learning to release the hurt allows us to move on with our lives.

After we release the resentment from the past through forgiveness, we must take care not to allow resentment to build up in the present or the future. As we let go of grudges, we no longer define life by how we've been hurt. Forgiveness is the vehicle through which we can find compassion and understanding for others and ourselves.

Affirmation Avenue

"Finally, brothers, whatever things are true, whatever things are honest, whatever things are just, whatever things are pure, whatever things are lovely, whatever things are of good report; if there be any virtue, and if there be any praise, think on these things." ~ Philippians 4:8

An affirmation is the act of declaring a positive statement or judgment to be true. Affirmations help us replace negative thoughts with more helpful life-enriching thoughts. By repeating affirmations for at least thirty days, you can recondition the mind to think about life in a positive way. I create my own affirmations but also like to read affirmations that have been written by others.

Whenever I come across relevant affirmations in my spiritual readings, I record them in my phone. Over the years, I have collected quite a few affirmations that help to raise my consciousness. If you think that you don't have time, recapture those long-lost wasted hours of surfing the Internet or watching TV. I was amazed by how much time I recaptured when I significantly reduced the amount of time I spent talking on the telephone. I take advantage of unoccupied time, like waiting in line at the store or in a traffic backup, to read and internalize affirmations. You can also place affirmations on your refrigerator, use them as a screensaver on your computer, or write them on your mirror or in a journal.

Listening to or reading positive literature each day also helps us to recondition the mind and improve our psyche, which ultimately improves our circumstances. I read something positive every morning when I awaken. I am in prayer during the morning, and I enjoy the solitude as I travel in my car. When I get to work, I read something else encouraging and uplifting. I try not to complain or associate with people who complain or talk about others, because this will only counteract the positive work that I am doing.

Creating Affirmations

To create an affirmation, make a list of the character traits that you desire. When creating your affirmations, write them in the present tense. The statements should be written with the ultimate result in mind. Louise Hay has a particularly good book on affirmations called *I Can Do It, How to Use Affirmations to Change Your Life*. This is an excellent way to learn about using affirmations correctly to improve virtually every aspect of your life. Reclaim the best possible health by affirming that every cell, organ, and function of the body performs optimally.

Repeat your affirmations in the morning and again in the evening for at least thirty days to internalize them as part of your psyche. When saying your affirmations, envision them as if they have already come to pass, and say them with feeling.

Sample Affirmations

I am radiantly and enthusiastically alive. I am whole and complete. I have perfect circulation, assimilation, and elimination. I am grateful for Divine health.

Today, I am divinely guided to do everything better. I now release all past negativity. I choose to feel safe, well, free and happy. Guilt, condemnation and blame no longer have any hold over me. I move into the light of my true being.

I am open and receptive to my true purpose in life. I am now willing to express all my gifts, talents, and abilities fully. I now release any restriction that I have placed on myself. I listen to my heart, and that which is for me to do reveals itself. I step into my ideal work. I live my vision and I am fulfilled.

I open myself to consider new ways to experience the amazing healing powers of my body. My body knows exactly what, when and how to do its work.

Visualization Voyage

There is nothing at all new, strange, or unusual about creative visualization. You are already using it every day, every minute, in fact. ~ Shakti Gawain

We consciously create a picture in our minds of something that we would like to experience. Performers and athletes who want to enhance their success use visualization. As Shakti Gawain says in the quote above, we are visualizing all the time. We are doing it unconsciously and are unaware that it is happening. We can easily determine what we are unconsciously visualizing by taking a good look at what is manifesting in our lives. If we are not happy with what is being produced, then we can consciously change what we see in our minds. Try visualization as a tool to create optimal health and ultimate wellness.

Visualization Exercise

Use the tool of visualization frequently in the quietness of the morning, upon awaking and before drifting off to sleep. Spend ten to fifteen minutes visualizing the things that you wish to accomplish in your lifetime. Create a movie of your life and see yourself accomplishing those things that you have always dreamed of, including perfect health, a great career, wonderful relationships, et cetera. Envision yourself healthy and physically fit. Concentrate your thoughts on desired outcomes and see yourself thankful for manifesting all your dreams. See yourself giving your friends high-fives for all your achievements.

Body Therapy

"Yet this is health: To have a body functioning so perfectly that when its few simple needs are met it never calls attention to its own existence." ~ Bertha Stuart Dyment

The body has a super-wisdom biased in favor of life rather than death. There is a universal tendency for everything to return to normal whenever the balance of life has been violated. The human body is always seeking to heal itself and is continuously giving us information. For example, when you cut your finger, your body will immediately begin healing itself. Everything in the human body can regenerate itself. The skin regenerates every twenty-eight days, the liver every six weeks, the kidneys every four weeks, and the bones every seven years.

Every statement that you make with deep feeling about your body, or any belief you hold about it has the potential to manifest. To promote healing, you must do more than just destroy a tumor because the genesis of a tumor takes years to develop and is only a symptom of a larger issue. The key to reversing illness in the body is transforming the imbalance in the mind, coupled with detoxifying the body and improving the body's internal resistance. This will bolster the immune system, which enhances the functioning of all cells. The body will heal itself if the process of change is maintained long enough for all the cells to change.

There are many healing practices used to promote balance throughout the human system. We can cater to the needs of our body and bring more balance into our lives with proper posture, diet, and exercise – the core of good health. Laughing and dancing are also very healing activities. Reconnective Healing® is believed to be one of the newest and most comprehensive forms of energetic healing currently available. Walking a labyrinth path is a way to quiet the mind, reduce stress and encourage insight and self-reflection. With proper treatment, nutrition, exercise, and perseverance, you can potentially guide your body to full health and recovery.

Body Boulevard
A Healthy Diet

Enough is as good as a feast. ~English Proverb

I have personally tried numerous fad diets. They all seemed to work for a time, but I eventually reached a plateau or returned back to my original weight. Then I discovered that my body craves what it needs and alerts me regarding the foods that I should avoid. For example, when I eat dairy products, they make me gaseous and bloated. I have a similar negative reaction to sugar, caffeine, crabmeat, spicy foods, soy products and meat. These foods are poisons that pollute my system. I feel sluggish, and find that I am extremely sensitive emotionally, whenever I indulge in these foods. I find that I feel more energetic and have a good mental outlook when I eat fruits, vegetables, beans, nuts and other healthy foods. I eat to live and prefer simple food, rather than the rich and spicy alternative.

Several of my unhealthy clients told me that they would not give up their favorite food even though they know that it is hurting their health, which may explain why obesity is the #2 cause of death in the United States. At the risk of unhealthy living, these people are happy as long as they can eat whatever foods they desire because they live to eat. You must pay closer attention to what your body is telling you if you want to achieve ultimate wellness. When your body gives you clues as to what foods are good for you and what you should stay away from, you should decipher the messages and make the appropriate decisions. The sooner that you take heed of the signals the better. The time to go to the doctor is when you first start noticing the lightheadedness or pain. If you are feeling discomfort, it is best not to wait for the heart attack or sugar coma before deciding to act.

Juice Feast

One of the alternative methods that I have used to heal my body is doing a Juice Feast. A Juice Feast is juicing an abundance of fresh organic fruits and vegetables to help to cleanse, heal and rebuild your body. Drinking only juice for a period of time is like eating on steroids because it rejuvenates your metabolism and digestive system. You get all the nutrients in liquid form, which are more easily assimilated by the body. Nutrients are also available to the body in much larger quantities than if the fresh produce was eaten whole, because juicing removes the indigestible fiber. When you eat a raw carrot, you are only able to assimilate about one percent of the available beta carotene because many of the nutrients are trapped in the fiber. When a carrot is juiced, removing the fiber, nearly one hundred percent of the beta carotene can be assimilated. Juicing gives your body a rest from digesting solid food. This is a natural way to remove waste matter trapped in the colon, which fosters the natural healing process.

Eating on a Raw Diet

Let me start off by saying that every diet does not work for everyone, so check with your doctor first and then listen to what your body is telling you. If some foods make you ill, then remove them from your diet. Conversely, if there are foods that make you feel good, then keep them as part of your diet.

Raw food has the best balance of water, nutrients, and fiber to meet your body's needs. Raw foods are easily digested, requiring only 24–36 hours for transit time through the digestive tract, as compared to 40–100 hours for cooked foods. Raw food is food that is not cooked above 118° Fahrenheit. It is believed that when food is cooked above this temperature many of the vitamins, minerals and protein are lost. Digesting cooked foods exhausts your body's energy and inhibits healing, decreases alertness, efficiency, and productivity. Cooked foods are said to suppress the immune system and causes the body to age prematurely. Eating live food has many benefits including an increase in energy and mental clarity, better sleep, and that you can eat as much as you want. In addition, raw foods increase regularity, and they are "green," so there's no packaging to recycle.

Over the years I have tried several diets, combining the best from each one. *Fit for Life* by Harvey and Marilyn Diamond are advocates of eating live...high-water-content food and encourage the consumption of raw fruits and vegetables. Fruits are best eaten fresh and raw, and since they do not require digestive juices, they should be eaten alone when possible. If they are eaten in combination with other food types, it may not allow other foods to be fully digested. The Diamonds also advise that fruit and fruit juice should be eaten from the time one awakes until noon because this is the time that our body is in the elimination cycle and fruits cleanse the body. All other foods should be eaten later in the day.

I have had the most success with combining the *Fit for Life* diet recommendations with *The Blood Type Diet* by Dr. Peter D'Adamo and *Beating Cancer with Nutrition* by Dr. Patrick Quillin. With these three diets, I learned that some foods are better for me than others. I only choose foods that have a medicinal value for my blood type and the highest benefit and nutrient density. I choose only the highest quality organic fruits, vegetables, nuts and seeds available. As a rule of thumb, the darker green the vegetable, the better. Lettuce and apples are considered the "junk-food" of produce.

Raw foods that score high for containing a wide range of cancer-fighting substances include grapes, blueberries, broccoli, cauliflower, cabbage, kale, spinach, romaine lettuce, beets, red cabbage, garlic, onions, scallions and tomatoes.

Eating raw is a personal experience and it does require that you explore what combinations work best for you. It's best to start the process of integrating more raw organic foods into your diet slowly. You can gradually begin to remove cooked foods and replace them with a raw equivalent. For the best results, keep your diet very simple and pre-plan your meals. I prepare my meals the night before and shop a little more often to ensure that I am getting the freshest produce possible.

Be careful about making eating a ritual or a religion. It is okay to eat what you want if it is in moderation. One of the things that I liked the most about *Fit for Life* is the "free day" where you can eat whatever you want one day each week (preferably the same day every week). This not only helps to keep you from craving or binging, but it helps to keep things interesting.

Physical Exercise

"The human body is a machine which winds its own springs." ~ Julien Offroy de la Mettrie

It took me many years to realize how important it is for me to deliberately move and stretch my body. When we sit in front of the TV or computer for hours on end, it slows down our metabolism, which results in increased weight, especially in our arms, thighs, and tummy. Our body needs to be stretched and exerted if we want to stay fit with toned muscles. Get in touch with what your body needs and become more aware of any stiffness or aches. To achieve your ideal weight, start a routine of walking up the steps instead of taking the elevator, or stretching to keep your body limber. Take your time and work your way up to some type of regular exercise routine or program that fits into your schedule. Some schools of thought recommend daily exercise, while others say to give the body a rest every other day. Do what you feel is right for you, but whatever you choose, the key is to remain consistent.

Laughing

A good laugh and a long sleep are the best cures in the doctor's book. ~ Irish Proverb

I am fortunate in that I had the opportunity to laugh a lot while I was growing up as a triplet. It was a lot of fun having two sisters who looked almost identical to me. My mother dressed us alike, and it was just like looking in the mirror all day. We used to laugh all day long. Sometimes we take ourselves way too seriously and laughing helps to keep you young and chipper. I still laugh out loud and find that I laugh at myself often.

Depending on the duration, laughter can be healing and uplifting. Laughter increases our serotonin level, which is a natural mood regulator. According to Paul E. McGhee, Ph.D., "Your sense of humor is one of the most powerful tools you have to make certain that your daily mood and emotional state support good health." Laughter also triggers healthy physical changes in your body. Humor and laughter strengthen your immune system, boost your energy, diminish pain, and protect you from the damaging effects of stress.

Norman Cousins, an adjunct professor of Medical Humanities for the School of Medicine at the UCLA, believed that human emotions were the key to human beings' success in fighting illness. He suffered from heart disease and developed a recovery program incorporating mega-doses of Vitamin C, along with a positive attitude, love, faith, hope, and laughter induced by watching Marx Brothers films. "I made the joyous discovery that ten minutes of genuine belly laughter had an anesthetic effect and would give me at least two hours of pain-free sleep,"

Cousins reported. Consider watching a good comedy show often to uplift and heal yourself with laughter.

Proper Rest

Even though I work hard and play hard, I make certain that I get the proper amount of rest. Gone are the nights of hanging out to the wee hours of the night and getting up to go to work the next morning. If I stay up late more than a few nights in a week, I will be sluggish, irritable, and dysfunctional. I need my rest to operate optimally. The amount of sleep that each person needs varies dramatically. Some need only a few hours, while others need ten to twelve hours. Listen to your body and give yourself the rest you need to look and feel your best.

Dancing

"Dance like no one is watching, love like you'll never be hurt, sing like no one is listening, and live like it's heaven on earth." ~ William Purkey

The National Heart, Lung and Blood Institute reports that dancing can lower your risk of coronary heart disease, decrease blood pressure, help you manage your weight and strengthen the bones of your legs and hips. I taught a life enrichment class at a local wellness center and met a beautiful woman with an awesome countenance. I noticed that there was something special about her and I connected with her energy immediately. I learned that she was a Neuromuscular Integrative Action

(NIA) dance instructor. NIA is a scientifically based fitness and healing system that blends aspects of martial arts, dance, and healing arts. She invited me to attend a dance class with her and I was pleasantly surprised by the experience. The powerful yet gentle movements of NIA allowed me to get in touch with the different parts of my body, which was phenomenally freeing and felt wonderful.

When I was a child, I remember doing the hokey pokey. It was a simple game where you would put various parts of your body in and out of a circle of children and then "shake it all about." I did the hokey pokey and did not care who was watching. I just did my thing. Somewhere between childhood and adulthood, I started to care about how others saw me when I danced. Now I recognize that dancing is just another way that we express our Divinity. So go ahead and give yourself permission to put on your favorite music and dance like nobody's watching. You will feel fantastic.

Reconnective Healing®
"The best and most efficient pharmacy is within your own system."
~ Robert C. Peale

I was invited to participate in a health fair at a Unity church in Washington, D.C. When I took a stroll through the room I met one of the other vendors who asked me if

I had ever heard about Reconnective Healing. I told her that I was not unfamiliar with this modality and then she asked me if I wanted to feel the energy. As she waved her hand around in a circular motion, I could feel a tingling in my hand that got stronger as she moved further away. Curious about how this could happen, I inquired how I could learn more. I was informed that training was available, but the next session was going to be held in Peru. This was a bit out of my reach, but I was so intrigued that I brought the book that she was selling called *Reconnective Healing: Heal Others, Heal Yourself* by Dr. Eric Pearl. I had several other books that I wanted to read at the time and that the book sat on my nightstand for months.

Several months later, I knew that it was time for me to resign from my job to do healing work full time. This created more time for me to do more research in the realm of healing. I remembered Dr. Pearl's book and began reading it at night before I went to bed. What I read astounded me and I could not believe what I was reading. Dr. Pearl stated this Reconnective energy was beginning to form in me as I was reading his book and he was right! My hands started tingling just as it did when I was at the health fair. How could this be?

I was so impressed by this discovery that I decided to go to the next training session that I could learn more about this Reconnective energy first-hand. The training was unlike anything that I had ever experienced in my life with each hour increasingly fascinating. I was so energized by what I learned during that class, that I extended my stay a few days to take The Reconnection® training.

I learned that Reconnective Healing® is a new broader spectrum of frequencies that have the capacity to bring about physical, mental, emotional, and spiritual healings. Dr. Eric Pearl discovered these frequencies in his chiropractic practice when his patients began reporting that they felt like they were being touched even though he hadn't physically touched them. Patients also reported seeing angels and receiving miraculous healings from cancers, AIDS-related diseases, Chronic Fatigue Syndrome, birth disfigurements, cerebral palsy, and other serious afflictions.

Reconnective Healing® is something that can be learned and is believed to be more expansive and comprehensive than other energy work like Reiki, Qi Gong or Acupuncture. Reconnective Healing® works differently than other energy healing techniques as it is composed of energy, light and information that allow the body to come back into balance so that you may heal yourself. Scientific studies suggest that these frequencies might even restructure our DNA, muscles, tissues and skeletal system, while at the same time balancing mental and emotional states.

Labyrinth Path

"Stand by the roads and look, And ask for ancient paths, where the good way is. And walk in it, and find rest for your souls." ~ Jeremiah 6:16

A friend from the spiritual center I attended was having a birthday and labyrinth walk celebration. The event sounded very interesting, and I decided to attend. When I arrived at her home, everyone was assembled in the backyard near a maze-like circular path that was patterned in the ground with grass and stones. We were instructed to follow the path and walk towards the center and then outwards again. We each took turns experiencing the peacefulness of the path. Intrigued by the experience, I decided to learn more about the practice of walking a labyrinth.

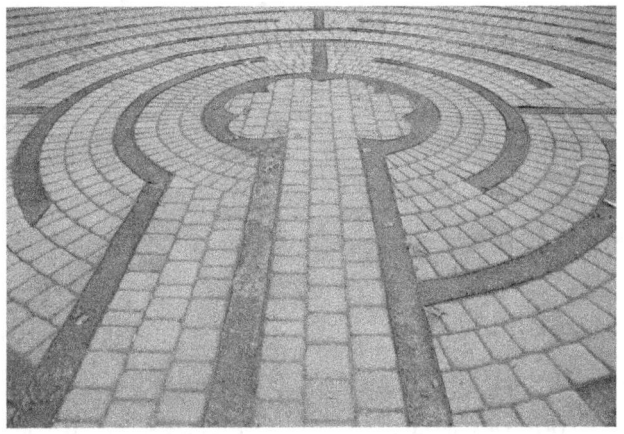

I discovered that a labyrinth is an ancient symbol that relates to healing and wholeness. It is found in traditions worldwide as a symbol that crosses cultural and religious boundaries. Most labyrinths are circular and have one thing in common: each has a path that begins on the perimeter and follows a winding and unobstructed route to the center.

The labyrinth is a complex circular path that is said to resemble our life's journey. As you walk the spiral pattern towards the center, one minute you are near the center and the next minute you are near the edge. The practice of labyrinth walking integrates the body with the mind and the mind with the soul. It sets the mind free by providing both a clear path and a safe peaceful environment.

Walking the labyrinth can bring solace through movement, and since the path is circuitous, both sides of the brain are engaged. As you walk from the circumference to the center, you may take this time to clear your mind. When you arrive at the center, open yourself to receive blessings and messages. As you return to the entrance of the labyrinth, this is when you can connect with a sense of healing and renewal.

Walking a labyrinth can be used as a prayer and walking meditation ritual. The labyrinth is a place to open your mind, listen to your heart and find renewal. It can be used for life balancing, stress releasing, enhancing creativity and fostering effective decision-making. To locate a labyrinth near you, search the Internet for Worldwide Labyrinth Locator.

Soul Therapy

"In my Soul there is a temple, a shrine, a mosque, a church that dissolves, that dissolves in God." ~ Rabia of Basra

Nurturing the soul enables us to take care of ourselves spiritually and increase our self-esteem. Dr. Wayne Dyer said, "Begin to see yourself as a soul with a body, rather than a body with a soul." Activities like prayer, meditation and journaling are a few ways to promote healing of the soul. Prayer is not just a matter of changing things externally, but one of working miracles in our inner nature. Meditation is a way to quiet the mind and create a sense of peacefulness. Journaling allows us to use ink and paper to express our feelings in an attempt to resolve life issues. Use these practices to create spiritual soil for balance, optimal healing, and ultimate wellness.

Prayer Place

"In prayer, it is better to have a heart without words than words without a heart."
~ Mahatma Gandhi

I am no stranger to the practice of prayer. My concept of prayer has gone through somewhat of a metamorphosis over the years. In the past, I only prayed when I was in desperate need of something. These were what you would call my "911 prayers." Then there were the times when I prayed my "Let's Make a Deal" prayer, promising God that I would exhibit a certain type of behavior if He would just give me the things that I wanted. All those years of begging and beseeching God did not yield the result that I sought. The truth is that God is not a wizard behind a curtain, doling out blessings to some and not to others.

According to *The Revealing Word,*

> "Prayer is communion between God and man.
> This communion takes place in the innermost
> part of man's being. It is the only way to cleanse
> and perfect the consciousness, and thus
> permanently heal the body."

Prayer conditions the mind to accept all the abundance that is already ours. The purpose of prayer is to reaffirm our union with the out-flowing giving-ness of life.

This reminds me of a song from the Unity church that helped me to put the power of prayer in perspective:

> Our thoughts are prayers and
> We are always praying.
> Our thoughts are prayers,
> Take charge of what you are saying.
> Seek a higher consciousness,
> A state of peacefulness,
> And know that God is always there.
> And every thought becomes a prayer.

The ancient Greek philosopher Epicurus said, "It is folly for a man to pray to the gods for that which he has the power to obtain by himself." It is better to appreciate what we already have than beg God for something we can manifest on our own. Our thoughts have creative power. Every prayer is answered by what we create with our mind, which manifests into the material world. Knowing what we want is the first step to achieving it. With active and conscious prayer, we can accomplish anything.

The MANTRA Project, a clinical trial of cardiac patients at Duke University, demonstrated the positive impact of prayer on patient outcomes, including fewer complications, less need for medication, and a quicker return to health.

One of the most powerful practices I learned from Religious Science is a unique five-step scientific method called a "Spiritual Mind Treatment." With this method of prayer, the first step is to recognize who God is in our lives. The next step is to unify with the One Mind and everything that exists. Then, we realize that which we desire is already done. Next, we give thanks for all of the good that flows through our life. The final step is to release the prayer to the Universe to bring about the manifestation of our desires. Praying in this manner has consistently attracted that which I desire into my life.

Sample Spiritual Mind Treatment

Step 1:

God is simply all that there is and God is good. God is the Creator of all things seen and unseen and is the source of all things.

Step 2:

I am one with God and connected to everything and everyone. There is no place where God is not because God is omnipresent. God is here with me in the here and now, and knows all that I am dealing with in my life at this time.

Step 3:

I am whole and see my body as healed from the top of my head to the soles of my feet. There is no sickness in God because God is perfect. I experience myself as a person who enjoys living a healthy lifestyle and a peaceful life.

Step 4:

I am thankful that this prayer is already answered and…

Step 5:

I release my word into the action of Universal Law knowing that it will attract unto me every good and perfect thing.

And so it is.

One of the keys to manifesting what we want is to pray with the attitude and feeling that we have already received the desired outcome. Pray out loud with faith and feeling, knowing that what you desire has already manifested, and you are merely conditioning the mind to see it in your reality. Pray from a place of knowing that all is done unto us as we believe and that one's word is the creative power of the universe. The law of attraction will match our belief, and you will see the result of your prayer to the extent that you believe it will come to fruition.

Meditation Lane

"Meditate not because you'll feel holy, but so you'll know that there's no difference between the times that you sit and the times that you don't." ~ Daniel Levin

Most of us have an inner landscape cluttered with incoherence as the mind leaps around in an undisciplined manner from one thing to another. Immature patterns of thought and feelings urge us here and there without our truly knowing what is going on. The goal of meditation is to be mindful and present in the moment. Here are some indications of a cluttered mind:

1. When you think the same thoughts that you've always thought even though they may no longer serve you.

2. When you dread doing something but do it anyway because you agreed to.

3. When you tell the same old victim story over and over for years.

4. When you are attached to things that you think define who you are.

5. When you worry.

6. When you do not accept and love yourself the way that you are.

When anxiety levels are elevated, meditation can offer a way to quiet the mind and help us to find peace. The purpose of meditating is to help us to get control of our thoughts. Meditation allows the mind to rest and accept inspiration. Slowing down our mind helps us to become more relaxed, which reduces stress and creates a peaceful countenance.

Evidence of the positive health-related results of meditation can be found in a clinical trial conducted by Kabat-Zinn, Lipworth, and Burney that examined the impact of mindful-meditations on ninety chronic pain patients. Significant reductions were reported in present-moment pain, psychological and other symptoms as well. A 2002 study by Keefer and Blanchard of patients with irritable bowel syndrome who meditated, determined that there were statistically significant reductions in their abdominal pain, and the changes were maintained over the long term.

One of the biggest challenges with meditation is learning to focus the mind. One way to slow down the number of thoughts going through the mind is to mentally focus on our breath as it flows through our nostrils. Release the thoughts that come in during meditation by opening a door and letting them out by either opening your mouth or by envisioning the thoughts going in one ear and out the other.

We are always thinking about some aspect of our lives and assimilating data. In this information-age we are often overwhelmed with avalanches of information continually bombarding us. Meditation provides the opportunity to slow things down and reduce our intake of information. We think that our accomplishments are manifested from what we are "doing," but it is the space between the thoughts where creation occurs. In *Getting in the Gap*, Dr. Wayne Dyer states, "It's the space between the notes that make the music, the space between the bars that holds the tiger."

There are as many ways to meditate as there are reasons to do so. If you have an active mind, you can meditate while you walk, run or during any other activity where you can focus and remain present in the moment. You can start this practice for a minute or two, and then work your way up to ten or twenty minutes at a time.

Practice, Practice, Practice

Catherine Ponder said that when you get your own thoughts and feelings in order, then the people and situations in your life respond in a more orderly way. I find that when I make time to meditate, the day goes along more smoothly. Although I have been practicing meditation for years, it often takes me ten to twenty minutes to quiet my mind, and even then, I am only able to focus my mind for a short period of time. Nevertheless, I make time each day to sit and be present with my breath and relax my body. Each time I am still, it is another opportunity for a "time out" for my mind and my body to unwind.

Meditation renews your energy and helps you to focus. Lao Tzu said, "Still and tranquility set things in order in the universe." Take time for yourself each day to get in touch with your Higher Power. Choose a meditation method that resonates with you the most and practice it daily until things in your life are set in order.

Journal Journey

"Journal writing is a voyage to the interior." ~Christine Baldwin

Journaling is the practice of keeping a diary that explores the thoughts and feelings surrounding the events of one's life. The purpose of journaling is to clarify what you are thinking and how you feel, to gain valuable self-knowledge. You can write about your feelings in detail as they relate to the stressful events you encounter. Journaling is also a good problem-solving tool, allowing you to hash out a problem and come up with solutions on paper. It is helpful to write out any thoughts that come to mind without partiality.

The health benefits of keeping a personal journal or diary have been proven. The pioneer of journal therapy, Dr. James W. Pennebaker, has been researching the effects of expressive writing for decades. He found that actively holding back feelings from others is extremely stressful. By simply expressing yourself through writing, you could potentially experience immediate life improvements. In addition, the well-being of your immune system is highly correlated with your psychological well-being. Stressful situations, such as exams, loneliness, divorce, or job loss can lead to adverse immunological changes. Similar to the effects of psychotherapy, journaling regularly can have a positive impact on the immune system. Simply writing about important experiences for as little as fifteen minutes per day not only reduce stress and anxiety, it can also lower heart rate, reduces pain, and reduce the need for medication. This is especially true if you write about traumatic life experiences and feelings.

Writing out negative situations helps us to process our feelings more fully by exploring and releasing the emotions involved. I always keep a composition notebook with me to write down feelings and ideas as they come to me. In the past, I used the dainty and decorative journals, but they were too restrictive, as I seemed to be more concerned about the amount of paper, I was using than fully recording my thoughts. Composition notebooks are inexpensive and give me plenty of room to write or draw, record my dreams, desires, affirmations. and notable events.

Space Therapy

"Space as the background invites existence, but is not singular. Space also accommodates the coordination of sense experience, the interconnection of objects, the substantiality of what exists, and the unifying of all physical appearance within a single matrix." ~ Tarthang Tulku

We must consider the effects of our environment because everything is energy connected in space, which has an impact on our mind, body and soul. All things in the universe are made up of either objects or space. Our personal energy manifests as a force in our homes and workplaces. These spaces also radiate an energy field or force which impacts us in some way, positively or negatively. To use an analogy of raisin bread, the bread represents the space, while the raisins represent the objects. As the bread holds the raisins in place, the energy of the space (bread) has an affect on the objects, and the objects (raisins) have a force on the space. If you remove the raisin, you will see an imprint of where the raisin was, but you will also see some of the bread residue on the raisin.

Feng Shui is one of the systems that we can use to foster an environment that supports our health and well-being. This ancient Chinese methodology helps us to understand the energetic vibrations of our space so that we can align with it to create harmony and balance. When the principles are followed correctly, they produce positive results in every area of our lives. When our homes or workspaces have negative energy or vibrations, they negatively impact us. A home with good energy has happy occupants that attract greater wealth, more loving and harmonious relationships, successful careers, and improved academic achievement.

There are also chemical, technological, and electromagnetic energies all around us that may be negatively affecting our health. If I told you that I knew about a way to prevent cancer, would you believe me? What you do not know about Geopathic Stress can kill you. It is my intention to share this information with as many people as possible so that they can protect themselves from this noxious energy.

Geopathic Stress is a medically accepted term for depleting earth energies caused by a disruption of the energy lines that are a part of the earth's own subtle energy field. These noxious earth energies are not visible, but they still influence a person's body, in a similar way that overexposure to radiation from x-rays causes cancer. When a person spends a considerable time in the zones influenced by such energies, their body becomes weakened and more susceptible to illness. We must learn to identify and neutralize these negative energies to allow the body to maintain its ultimate state of health.

Feng Shui Way

"If there is light in the soul, there is beauty in the person. If there is beauty in the person, there is harmony in the house. If there is harmony in the house, there is order in the nation. If there is order in the nation, there will be peace on earth."
~Old Chinese Proverb

After reading Eckhart Tolle's book, *The Power of Now*, I became more aware that there is more space than anything else, and it only appears that there are more objects because that is what we are focusing on. Later, I was guided to the art of Feng Shui and was amazed by the subtle but powerful ways that we interact with our surroundings. Using what I learned, I began adjusting my space to support the inner healing work that I was doing, achieving noteworthy results. I felt better, and the negative situations in my life began to improve. My home was more comfortable and arranged in a way that felt supportive and nurturing.

Everything is energy vibrating at different levels and our whole cosmos is based on the flow of energy. Feng Shui is a system of principles that can be used to assess the condition of a space. These systems help us to interpret the story that our environment is telling us and provides ways to energetically align and tune our surroundings to a nurturing frequency. Feng Shui teaches us an awareness and sensitivity of how an environment feels, and how to maximize the harmony within our space. For areas that are out of alignment with universal energy there are remedies to correct deficiencies. There are also treatments to enhance the positive environmental attributes.

In her book, *Healing Design*, Hope Karan Gerecht refers to three main tenants of Feng Shui:

> (1) to elevate our life by encouraging the flow of vital energy (chi) in our living environments, (2) to deflect unfortunate energy (sha); and (3) to create balance in our home environment...

The intrinsic benefit of Feng Shui principles is that they offer support in our relationships, economic outlook, mental stability, education, career, and health. As increased and balanced energy meanders gently through our environments, we experience better health, enhanced creativity, a deeper spiritual connection, more rewarding relationships, stronger career support, and increased prosperity.

It is said that our home is like a mirror of our life. Feng Shui uses metaphors, associations, and symbolism to help us determine how our space impacts our existence. Colors, position, energy movement and the very items in our possession have a peculiar way of altering our mood, character, and potential. Feng Shui is based on two premises, the first being that a person's state of mind energetically affects his environment for good or ill; the second is that the condition of the environment affects man's internal state. Using Feng Shui, we can align the energy in our space in such a way that good energy nurtures and supports us.

In her book, *The Western Guide To Feng Shui*, Terah Kathryn Collins wrote a story to illustrate how our environment can negatively impact our health:

> A man has to stoop under an overgrown branch to get in his front door. He does not trim the branch and has to stoop every day for a year to get in his door. Soon, he begins to walk in a stooped posture everywhere he goes. One branch in need of a trim has changed this man's gait. His stoop leads to illness, loss of work, and financial problems.

Had the man known about Feng Shui, his illness could have been easily circumvented by simply pruning the tree.

Our environment reveals the thoughts that could be contributing to our illnesses and dissatisfaction. Symbolically speaking, there is an anatomical association between the different parts of the body and the areas in our homes. A problem in a particular area of the home could indicate a problem in the corresponding part of our body/life and vice-versa.

On the pages that follow, you will find a few ways to apply Feng Shui principles to your life: Cleansing, Clutter-Free, Attracting More Love and Increasing Wealth.

Cleansing

One of the ways that you can apply Feng Shui to heal your life is by "cleansing" your space. Just as the surfaces of furniture collect dust and dirt, our space collects negative energy that does not support us. A home that has had a death, years of arguing, a divorce, or unhappiness, carries a residue of negative energy long after the occupants have moved out. Cleansing a space removes unwanted negative energy, allowing good energy to flow. We can cleanse an area by burning bundled or dried sage, using sound (chimes or singing bowls), burning incense, or doing a spring cleaning with the intention of removing unwanted stagnant energy.

Clutter-Free

Another fundamental Feng Shui principle that is conducive to good health is the necessity to keep your space clutter-free. We talked earlier about the practice of meditation to clear the mind. There is a subtle relationship between physical and spiritual clutter, which may reveal a mentality of lack. Clearing up physical clutter helps to clear the mind. Clutter is related to instincts of self-protection, leading to hoarding on the one hand and to feelings of insecurity on the other.

It is important to note that my clients who had lots of clutter in their homes also suffered from a major ailment or disease. When there is clutter or negative energy, our outlook and health deteriorate. Even small amounts of clutter have negative impacts and subconsciously make us feel that there is something left undone. An area with too many papers, books or unused items can make us feel uneasy and in a state of constant irritation. Here are some easy ways to determine what to release:

1. Items that you do not need but just can't get rid of.

2. Items that you do not use but are holding onto.

3. Items that you cannot let go of because you fear you won't be able to purchase them again.

If you are having difficulty releasing the clutter in your space, ask yourself the following questions:

1. Have I used this item in the last six months?

2. Can someone else make better use of this item?

3. Does this item bring me happiness or make me feel good?

When we are willing to release old or worn-out possessions, we make room for new, exciting, and refreshing items and experiences. We get a new lease on life and everything begins to flow.

Attracting More Love

The wonderful thing about Feng Shui is the many ways that you can attract more love into your life. When I arrive at the homes of my female clients, invariably I find them filled with pictures or artworks of women who are alone, unhappy, or distorted in some way. Artwork in the home should represent a balance of male and female energy. It should also be representative of the lifestyle you desire. Homes dominated by artwork that are contradictory to the kind of person you are seeking could have a negative effect on your chances of attracting a mate. It is not recommended that you place pictures of single people unless you want to reinforce that relationship status. By maintaining a balance of male and female décor and hanging pictures of loving couples to symbolize love and commitment, you increase your chances of attracting like energy. Take a look around your space to gauge the predominant energy of the artwork in your home.

Increasing Wealth

The most enticing aspect of Feng Shui is the amazing impact it can have on "money luck." Feng Shui can be designed to focus on creating wealth, prosperity, and abundance. When your home, workplace or office is oriented to bring about good Feng Shui, income usually increases. When you place money symbols in the far left hand corner of a room or home, it activates wealth energy and is said to attract wealth opportunities. A few months after I performed a Feng Shui consultation for a song writer, he was receiving large checks. As luck would have it, a well-known musician was looking for new material. Out of all of the millions of songs that could have been chosen, the artist picked one of my client's songs that was written twenty years earlier. Now my client is living very comfortably and enjoying the finer things in life.

The space that surrounds us should not be overlooked as a force to be reckoned with. Feng Shui is not just about becoming wealthy or achieving success – it is concerned with enriching lives, reducing aggravation, and bringing happiness into relationships. Feng Shui is a system of principles that helps us to maintain a good energy flow in our surroundings, resulting in balance and harmony in our lives. The advantage of using Feng Shui is the positive benefit it creates for everyone. It is about feeling happy, prosperous and contented.

Geopathic Stress Crossing – Prevent Heart Disease and Cancer

"Most of the objects found in nature emit stable frequencies… Humans are the only creatures that have the capacity to resonate with all other creatures and objects found in nature… We can give out energy and also receive energy in return." ~ Dr. Masaru Emoto

In my work as a Holistic Spatial Therapist, I combine the principles of Feng Shui with the science of neutralizing negative earth radiation such as Geopathic Stress. Geopathic Stress occurs when underground streams, sewers, water pipes, electricity, tunnels, subways, mineral formations, and geological faults distort the earth's electromagnetic field. Electro-magnetic frequencies are caused by the overuse of electricity, including microwaves, cell phones, cell phone towers, power lines and transformer boxes. Together they form a wave or fog of negative energy that surrounds us. These energies combine with natural earth frequencies to form a curtain above and below the earth. These types of energies are unavoidable, particularly in a city. It is probable that a person living in a heavily populated area will have an increased risk of developing cancer due to these negative earth energies.

There have been reports of health improvements from the owners of homes where the negative earth energy was neutralized. I personally dropped twelve pounds because my immune system no longer had to work so hard to protect me from the harmful low-level radiation that was affecting the space in my home. One client, an elderly woman in her seventies, was on nine medications and suffered from fluctuating blood pressure, diabetes, arterial fibrillation, high cretin levels, high pulse rate, severe headaches, kidney problems, digestive system problems, back problems, and fatigue. Within months after I performed spatial therapy in her home, we were both astonished and happy to hear that her health reports began showing consistent improvement. The doctors were baffled and told her that they have never seen this type of a turn-around. Each doctor gave her a clean bill of health and she was eventually able to stop taking seven of the nine medications she relied on before the session and has continued to have good health ever since.

We are living in an environment where we are bombarded with so much electromagnetic energy that our bodies are unable to adapt. The National Institute of Environmental Health Sciences reported a link between exposure to electro-magnetic fields and certain site-specific cancers, namely leukemia and central nervous system lymphomas. In her book, *Earth Radiation*, Kathe Bachler presented a scientific study of eleven thousand people in over three thousand apartments, houses, and workplaces in fourteen countries. The astonishing results revealed that sleeping or sitting in areas with Geopathic Stress was found to be a common factor in many serious and/or long-standing illnesses, such as cancer, heart disease, migraines, sudden infant death, poor school performance, unwanted behavior, and psychological conditions.

The human body operates according to very complex electrochemical processes, which can be easily disturbed by Geopathic Stress. These negative energies lower our immune system and adversely affect our cellular structure. Alterations in our biological functioning can lead to adverse health effects. If sleep patterns are disturbed, not only can this make us feel tired and irritable, but it can also produce a litany of more serious illnesses over time. The body's resistance to viruses and bacteria can become affected when the natural rhythms within the body are constantly distorted during sleep. But we are not powerless against these negative effects. We can take control of our health by learning to neutralize these energies in our homes for ourselves, our families, and by sharing this knowledge with our communities.

Treatment for Geopathic Stress is well accepted in Europe as practitioners work together with doctors to not only treat the symptoms of the illness but oversee the patient's lifestyle and psychological well-being. In the United States, treatment for Geopathic Stress is virtually non-existent; it is my vision to share the technique of Holistic Spatial Therapy with the millions of people who suffer from chronic illness unnecessarily and to those who want to prevent debilitating attacks on their health. To lessen the effects of man-made stresses in our homes, we must reduce the amount of electro-magnetic fields, pollution and clutter. We can also neutralize negative earth radiation to achieve increased energy, better sleep quality and to boost our immunity.

Thousands of people have benefited from clearing their property of Geopathic Stress and have experienced improvements in finances, health, and relationships almost immediately. Anyone can learn the skills and obtain the tools necessary to neutralize these energies and teach others to do the same. The techniques are simple and relatively inexpensive, in comparison to the cost of managing a chronic illness. Sessions generally only take a few hours to produce positive results.

There's No Place Like Home

In the final act of *The Wizard of Oz*, it is revealed that the Wizard is an imposter. He cleverly granted the Scarecrow, the Lion, and the Tin Man's wishes for healing their defects by showing them they already had the qualities within themselves the entire time they were seeking them. In all three cases, they thought they lacked something – intellect (Mind), courageous strength (Body), and a sensitive heart (Soul) respectively – but they were only unaware of the power that resided within. It became increasingly evident that they each had the qualities inside of them as their adventures progressed.

Dorothy's wish was to return home to Kansas (Space). At the conclusion of the film, Glinda, the Good Witch, explains to Dorothy that she had the power to fulfill her dream of returning home all along. The ruby slippers that she had given to Dorothy at the beginning of the story were the key that would take her there. Glinda did not tell Dorothy about the power of the slippers earlier on because she wanted Dorothy to learn that she didn't need to run away from home to find her heart's desire. After Dorothy says a tearful goodbye to the friends she met in Oz, she follows Glinda's instructions to close her eyes, tap her heels together three times and chant, "There's no place like home." When she does this, the magical Land of Oz disappears and Dorothy arrives back in her hometown, in her own bed, as if all her adventures in Oz were a dream.

We were all born with the power to heal ourselves and it is part of our DNA. This gift has always been available and always will be. We can call on it at will and use our inner awareness to create miracles. Healing is a process, and we must be willing to do the work required to bring about the changes we seek. If we want our experiences to be different, then we must be willing to do something different. Daydreaming, hoping, wishing, and longing are not the avenues that bring about transformation. It takes dedication, perseverance, courage and sometimes traveling the road less traveled.

We can take charge of our healing by changing how we feel about our lives. Good energy flows more easily when we feel good. When we are feeling nervous, irritable, sad, confused, or hurt, we must pay closer attention to the thoughts we are thinking that are causing those feelings, and then choose to think thoughts that help us feel better. Healthy feelings lead to a healthy life. This is how we heal ourselves from the inside out.

Just as Dorothy's journey concluded once she returned home, the conclusion of our own journey to ultimate wellness may very well end in our own homes as well. By utilizing Feng Shui principles and Geopathic Stress neutralization techniques, we can finally address the root cause of chronic illnesses or persistent psychological conditions while creating a nurturing and supportive environment to help us reach fulfillment in all areas of our lives.

While we each must take responsibility for our own experience and the development of our consciousness, let us not forget that we are also a part of a collective experience. Dorothy had the company of three friends on her journey to the Land of Oz, and they all supported one another. One of the greatest contributions that we can make in our world is to be aware of the kind of energy that we are contributing to the collective consciousness. Simply put, our thoughts are either creating health or creating illness for ourselves and the world. Eckhart Tolle said, "The world can only change from within." It is my wish that we each begin to consistently think healthy and peaceful thoughts for ourselves and for others, so that we can create the ultimate wellness that we all want and crave.

There are millions of people who could benefit from learning alternative ways to heal and support themselves. It can be very satisfying to help those closest to us become healthier and more fulfilled. Please consider sharing the ideas or concepts that you found helpful with a friend or family member who may be inspired by them.

I am thankful for the opportunity to share this life-giving information with you, and I am extremely blessed to have spent this time with you in spirit. I hope that you discovered something that will set you on the path of healing your mind, body, soul, and surrounding space. Jesus is most remembered for the many miracles he performed including healing the sick, helping the blind to see, the deaf to hear, turning water into wine and feeding the multitude. We must also remember that he said, "Greater works shall ye do."

It is my intention to liberate millions of people from unnecessary pain and suffering by educating the public about a holistic approach to wellness. I am clear that this is my purpose for being on the planet. I invite you to join me in creating this global shift and make miracles happen.

About the Author

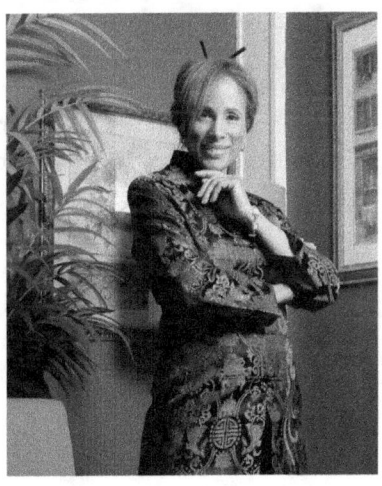

"The doctor of the future will give no medicine but will interest his patients in the care of the human frame, in diet, and in the cause and prevention of disease." ~Thomas Edison

Renée Alleyne, Ph.D. also known as Dr. Renée is an author, speaker and holistic life coach specializing in simple ways to prevent and heal chronic illness. Her mission is to empower women to live the life of their dreams.

Dr. Renée is the creator of the Wellness Makeover Program, which helps women to create a wellness formula that addresses root causes rather than cure symptoms. She received her doctoral degree in Holistic

Life Coaching from the University of Sedona, International Metaphysical Ministry.

A channel for healing, Dr. Renée provides Reconnective Healing®, which activates your healing potential with information, energy, and light. She is also certified to perform The Reconnection®, which helps you to accelerate and fulfill your purpose for being the planet.

Dr. Renée is proficient at clearing negative earth radiation from your space, which has been proven to be the root cause of many chronic illnesses like cancer and heart disease. For more information, please visit DrRenee.com, or e-mail: Book@DrRenee.com.

Acknowledgements

Anyone who has written a published work knows that it is a major undertaking. I would like to express deep gratitude to the people who helped me along the way to make this book a reality:

Rev. Dr. LaVerne Adams (Editorial Support)

Windy Blount (Hair Stylist)

Alexandra Escudero (Editorial Support)

Tonika Garibaldi (Photographer, Labyrinth)

Phrizbie Design (Illustrations)

Style in a Nutshell, Chris Loney (Fashion Stylist)

Kaye Love (Editorial Consultant)

Tamika Pickney (Makeup Artist)

Leslie Monroe (Editorial Support)

Janice Riley (Editorial Support)

Billy Wilkins (Consultant)

Paulette Williams (Inspirational Support)

L.T. Woody (Editorial Advisor)

Coaching, Consulting, Wellness
Retreats & Regimens

For the latest information go to www.DrRenee.com.